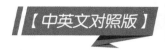

新型冠状病毒肺炎肺部CT表现特点及演变过程

COVID-19 Pulmonary CT Features and Evolution

季文斌　主编

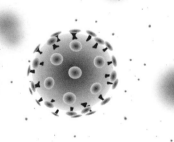

科学技术文献出版社
SCIENTIFIC AND TECHNICAL DOCUMENTATION PRESS

·北京·

图书在版编目（CIP）数据

新型冠状病毒肺炎肺部CT表现特点及演变过程：汉英对照 / 季文斌主编 . —北京：科学技术文献出版社，2020.8

书名原文：COVID-19 Pulmonary CT Features and Evolution

ISBN 978-7-5189-6659-2

Ⅰ . ①新… Ⅱ . ①季… Ⅲ . ①日冕形病毒—病毒病—肺炎—计算机X线扫描体层摄影—研究—汉、英 Ⅳ . ① R563.104

中国版本图书馆 CIP 数据核字（2020）第 063345 号

新型冠状病毒肺炎肺部 CT 表现特点及演变过程（汉英对照）

策划编辑：张　蓉　责任编辑：彭　玉　张　波　责任校对：王瑞瑞　责任出版：张志平		

出　版　者　科学技术文献出版社

地　　　址　北京市复兴路15号　邮编100038

编　务　部　（010）58882938，58882087（传真）

发　行　部　（010）58882868，58882870（传真）

邮　购　部　（010）58882873

官 方 网 址　www.stdp.com.cn

发　行　者　科学技术文献出版社发行　全国各地新华书店经销

印　刷　者　北京地大彩印有限公司

版　　　次　2020年8月第1版　2020年8月第1次印刷

开　　　本　889×1194　1/32

字　　　数　180千

印　　　张　6.875

书　　　号　ISBN 978-7-5189-6659-2

定　　　价　68.00元

主编简介

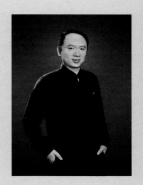

季文斌
主任医师，教授，硕士研究生导师。台州恩泽医疗中心（集团）放射学部主任，浙江省台州医院放射科主任。

社会任职

浙江省医师协会放射学分会常务委员、浙江省生物医学工程学会放射专委会常务委员、浙江省放射学分会委员、浙江省医学介入分会委员、浙江省抗癌协会介入分会委员。

专业特长

主要从事放射诊断与综合介入工作，擅长各类肿瘤的早期诊断、肿瘤影像综合评价，专注于分子影像学研究工作。

所获奖项

主办国家继续教育项目1项，省级继续教育项目1项；主持省部级科研项目3项，厅局级科研项目4项；获厅局级科技奖2项。

主要作品

近五年以第一作者或通讯作者在*Radiology*等杂志发表论文共11篇，其中新型冠状病毒肺炎相关论文2篇；主编出版专著2部。

编委会

序

2019年年底，一场新型冠状病毒感染的肺炎疫情在武汉暴发，并且随着春节返乡的人群向其他省份扩散，浙江台州也成了疫情的高发区之一。

台州恩泽医疗中心（集团）第一时间肩负起抗击疫情的重任，以过硬的医疗技术投入抗击新型冠状病毒肺炎的战役中。台州恩泽医疗中心（集团）放射学部季文斌主任团队在新型冠状病毒肺炎的CT诊断、治疗效果评价等方面取得很好的专业成果。2020年2月初，他们在国际顶尖的放射学期刊*Radiology*上发表了2篇关于新型冠状病毒肺炎CT诊断的论文，介绍了对新型冠状病毒肺炎CT诊断的经验。现在，他们又整理、完成了《新型冠状病毒肺炎肺部CT表现特点及演变过程》一书，把他们的宝贵经验奉献给大家。当前，我国在抗击新型冠状病毒肺炎疫情方面已经取得阶段性的胜利。但是，病毒没有国界，新型冠状病毒肺炎目前正在其他国家肆虐，威胁着成千上万人的生命安全。美国、意大利、西班牙等国的新型冠状病毒肺炎发病人数与死亡人数均远远超过我们国家。我相信季文斌主任团队主编的《新型冠状病毒肺炎肺部CT表现特点及演变过程》一书将为这些抗击新型冠状病毒肺炎的国家带来重要的参考价值。

我们的时代是迅猛发展的时代，是团结奋进的时代，是新人辈出的时代。青出于蓝而胜于蓝，看到季文斌取得的成绩，作为他的导师，我感到由衷的高兴！希望台州恩泽医疗中心（集团）和季文斌主任团队继续努力，并祝愿他们取得更加丰硕的成果！

浙江大学医学院附属邵逸夫医院

车士正

2020年4月10日

Preface

A sudden outbreak of 2019 novel coronavirus pneumonia (COVID-19) occurred in Wuhan in late 2019, and spreaded to other provinces as people returned home from Wuhan during the Spring Festival. Therefore, Taizhou, Zhejiang province has become one of the high-epidemic areas.

Taizhou Enze Medical Center is the first to shoulder the responsibility of fighting COVID-19 with strong medical technology. Wenbin Ji, director of radiology department of Taizhou Enze Medical Center, has made excellent professional achievements in CT diagnosis and treatment effect evaluation of COVID-19. At the beginning of February 2020, two papers on CT diagnosis for COVID-19 were published in *Radiology,* a leading international radiology journal, to introduce their experience in the CT diagnosis for COVID-19. Now, they have compiled and completed the book *COVID-19 Pulmonary CT Features and Evolution*, which brings their valuable experience to the public. At present, China's fight against the COVID-19 epidemic has achieved a phased victory. But the virus has no borders, and COVID-19 is currently raging in other countries around the world, threatening the lives of thousands of people.

The number of COVID-19 cases and deaths in the United States, Italy, Spain, and other countries are far larger than those in our country. I believe that the book *COVID-19 Pulmonary CT Features and Evolution*, edited by director Wenbin Ji's team, will be of important reference value to these countries fighting against the novel coronavirus pneumonia.

Our era is an era of rapid development, an era of solidarity, and an era of new generations. The pupil learns from and outdoes his teacher. As his tutor, I feel very glad to see the achievements he has made! I hope Taizhou Enze Medical Center and director Wenbin Ji's team continue to work hard and achieve more fruitful results!

Sir Run Run Shaw Hospital affiliated to Zhejiang University
Shizheng Zhang
4,10[th], 2020

前 言

　　新型冠状病毒肺炎于2019年年底被发现，目前在全球蔓延，该病发展速度较快，且主要累及肺部，在肺部CT上有特征性表现。台州恩泽医疗中心（集团）收治了145例新型冠状病毒肺炎患者，其中既有危重症患者，亦有普通型患者，而且这145例患者均有完整的影像资料。鉴于此，我们编撰了《新型冠状病毒肺炎肺部CT表现特点及演变过程》一书，并做成中英文对照版，期望给正处于抗击新型冠状病毒肺炎的医务工作者提供一些经验。

　　本书首先从新型冠状病毒肺炎的发展历程、流行病学、感染机制、病原学及CT检测价值等方面阐述了新型冠状病毒肺炎的整体情况。继而从临床表现、临床分期、检查流程、诊断规范、影像分期及病理基础等方面阐述了新型冠状病毒肺炎的肺部影像学检查基础与规范。再重点分析肺部CT各期的表现特点，这一部分以丰富且典型的肺部CT图片详细介绍了病变初期、进展期、高峰期及消散期的特征性表现。我们希望通过肺部CT图片来诠释新型冠状病毒肺炎的CT诊断经验，希望读者能从中得到一些启发与感悟。同时感谢我的导师章士正教授为本书作序！

本书的出版汇聚了全体编写人员的心血，也离不开医院的大力支持，在此表示由衷的感谢！由于我们的经验有限，不完善之处在所难免，请各位读者批评指正。

台州恩泽医疗中心（集团）

2020年4月10日

Foreword

COVID-19 has spread around the world since it has been discovered in 2019. It develops rapidly and mainly involves the lungs and has its characteristic manifestations on chest CT. Taizhou Enze Medical Center has treated 145 cases of COVID-19 with a complete image data, among which there are critical cases and common cases. In view of this, we have compiled the book *COVID-19 Pulmonary CT Features and Evolution* and made into a English-Chinese bilingual version, to provide experience in the chest CT diagnosis for the medical staff who are currently fighting against COVID-19.

First of all, this book describes the overall situation of novel coronavirus pneumonia in terms of its development history, epidemiology, infection mechanism, etiology and CT detection value. Secondly, the author expounds the basis and standard of pulmonary imaging examination of the novel coronavirus on the basis of its clinical manifestations, clinical staging, examination process, diagnostic criteria, image staging and pathological basis. And then focuses on the analysis of lung CT features of each stage, in this part, rich and typical CT images are used to introduce the initial stage, progression stage, peak period and dissipation stage of the lesions. We hope to interpret the CT diagnosis experience of COVID-19 through lung CT images, and hope that readers can get some inspiration and insights from it. At the same time, I would like to thank my tutor Professor Shizheng Zhang for writing the foreword for this book!

The publication of this book brings together the painstaking efforts of all the writers, and cannot do without the strong support of the hospital! I would like to express my sincere thanks here. Due to our limited experience in this book, the imperfections are inevitable, please criticize and correct.

Taizhou Enze Medical Center

Wenbin Ji

4,10[th], 2020

目　录

CONTENTS

1

第一章

新型冠状病毒肺炎概论

第一节　新型冠状病毒肺炎的发现与发展历程

2020 年 1 月 7 日，实验室检测出一种新型冠状病毒，并获得该病毒的全基因组序列。经核酸检测共检测出新型冠状病毒阳性结果 15 例，从 1 例阳性患者样本中分离出该病毒，其在电镜下呈典型的冠状病毒形态。同日，专家组认为，武汉不明原因的病毒性肺炎病例的病原体初步判定为新型冠状病毒。

2020 年 1 月 20 日，国家卫生健康委员会（简称国家卫健委）发布 2020 年第 1 号公告，将新型冠状病毒感染的肺炎纳入《中华人民共和国传染病防治法》规定的乙类传染病，并采取甲类传染病进行预防和控制。将新型冠状病毒感染的肺炎纳入《中华人民共和国国境卫生检疫法》规定的检疫传染病。

2019 年 12 月 31 日，中国报告了湖北省武汉市的一组肺炎病例，最终确认了一种新型冠状病毒。

2020 年 1 月 11 日，武汉出现首例死亡患者，该患者曾持续暴露于华南海鲜市场，在持续 7 天发烧、咳嗽和呼吸困难的情况下入院治疗。

2020 年 2 月 7 日，国家卫健委发出通知，决定将"新型冠状病毒感染的肺炎"暂命名为"新型冠状病毒肺炎"，简称"新冠肺炎"，英文名称为"Novel Coronavirus Pneumonia"，简称"NCP"。

2020 年 2 月 22 日，国家卫健委官方网站发布"关于修订新型冠状病毒肺炎英文命名事宜的通知"，决定将"新型冠状病毒肺炎"英文名称修订为"COVID-19"，与世界卫生组织命名保持一致。

2020 年 1 月 31 日，世界卫生组织建议将当前新型冠状病毒肺炎暂命名为"2019-nCoV acute respiratory disease"，把病毒暂命名为"2019-nCoV"，"2019"代表"首次出现的年份"，"n"表示"novel（新）"，"CoV"表示"Coronavirus（冠状病毒）"。

2020 年 2 月 11 日，世界卫生组织总干事谭德塞（Tedros Adhanom Ghebreyesus）在瑞士日内瓦宣布，将新型冠状病毒感染的肺炎命名为"COVID-19"，其中"CO"代表"corona（冠状物）"，"VI"代表"virus（病毒）"，"D"代表"disease（疾病）"。同日，国际病毒分类委员会（International Committee on Taxonomy of Viruses，ICTV）将新型冠状病毒命名为 SARS-CoV-2。ICTV 冠状病毒研究小组在生物学预印本网站 BioRxiv 上发表的论文强调了 SARS-CoV-2 与 SARS 病毒的相似性。

2020 年 4 月 14 日 6 时，全球新型冠状病毒肺炎累计确诊病例超过 190 万例，达到 1 912 923 例，累计死亡 119 212。美国累计确诊 583 870 例，累计死亡 23 485。西班牙累计确诊 169 628 例，死亡 17 628 例。意大利累计确诊 159 516 例，死亡 20 465 例。除美国外，法国、英国和土耳其单日新增病例均超过 4000 例，新增确诊患者数量最多。

2020 年 3 月 8 日，海外累计确诊 25 561 例，其中治愈 2730 例，死亡 501 例。海外在治的病例数（22 330）已经超过中国（20 611），而且还在快速增长中。

2020 年 3 月 6 日，欧洲疫情暴发，据法国欧洲时报社报道，截至巴黎时间 3 月 5 日 20 时，欧洲地区累计报告新型冠状病毒感染病例 5843 例，相比 3 月 5 日 8 时增加 1347 例。其中，意大利当日增加 769 例，总例数增至 3858 例；德国当日增加 169 例，总例数增至 547 例；法国当日增加 138 例，总例数增至 423 例。

2020 年 3 月 19 日，意大利死亡人数已超中国，感染人数达 41 035 例；美国的感染人数也已超过 10 000 万例。

第二节　新型冠状病毒肺炎的流行病学

一、冠状病毒的概念

冠状病毒在系统分类上属套式病毒目、冠状病毒科、冠状病毒属。冠状病毒属是一类具有囊膜、基因组为线性单股正链的 RNA 病毒，在自然界广泛存在。同时也是家畜、宠物，甚至人类疾病的重要病原，可引起多种急慢性疾病。呼吸系统感染是冠状病毒对人类的主要影响之一。

由于冠状病毒对温度很敏感，在 33 ℃时生长良好，但在 35 ℃时会受到抑制。因此，冬季和早春是该病毒感染疾病的流行季节。同时，冠状病毒也是成年人普通感冒的主要病原之一，儿童感染率较高，主要是上呼吸道感染，一般很少波及下呼吸道。另外，该病毒还可引起婴幼儿急性肠胃炎，主要症状是水样便、发热、呕吐，严重者甚至出现血水样便，极少数情况下也可引起神经系统综合征。

2019-nCoV 是目前已知的第七种可以感染人的冠状病毒，其余 6 种分别是 HCoV-229E、HCoV-OC43、HCoV-NL63、HCoV-HKU1、SARS-CoV（引发重症急性呼吸综合征）和 MERS-CoV（引发中东呼吸综合征）。2019-nCoV 是一种新出现的病原体，具有传染性强、传播速度快等特点。2019-nCoV 引发的疾病既不是流行性感冒，也不是 SARS。

二、新型冠状病毒肺炎的流行现状

截至 2020 年 2 月 21 日 24 时，全国 31 个省（自治区、直辖市）和新疆生产建设兵团报告，累计确诊病例 53 284 例（其中重症病例 11 477 例），累计治愈出院病例 20 659 例，累计死亡病例 2345 例，累计报告确诊病例 76 288 例，现有疑似病例 5365 例，累计追踪到密切接触者 618 915 人，尚在医学观察的密切接触者 113 564 人。湖北省累计治愈出院病例 13 557

例（其中武汉 7206 例），累计死亡病例 2250 例（其中武汉 1774 例），累计确诊病例 63 454 例（其中武汉 45 660 例）。

截至 2020 年 2 月 21 日，韩国新增新型冠状病毒肺炎确诊病例 100 例，累计确诊 204 例；日本累计确诊病例 728 例，其中有死亡病例 3 例；美国疾病控制与预防中心（Centers for Disease Control and Prevention，CDC）确认，美国境内已确诊 34 例新型冠状病毒肺炎病例。

截至 2020 年 3 月 30 日，西班牙卫生部确认有 12 298 名医务人员新型冠状病毒检测结果呈阳性。同日，意大利国家高等卫生研究院发布数据：意大利医务人员感染新型冠状病毒的人数共计 8358 例，相比前一天上升 595 例，因感染新型冠状毒病去世的医师达 63 人。

截至北京时间 2020 年 3 月 20 日 11 时，全球新型冠状病毒肺炎确诊病例累计 244 421 例，死亡病例 10 027 例，死亡人数破万。自疫情暴发近 3 个月以来，全球已有近 25 万人感染新型冠状病毒，病毒已蔓延至除南极洲以外的所有大陆。目前，中国疫情快接近尾声，欧洲、伊朗和美国的疫情却日益严峻，7 个国家的确诊人数突破 1 万。

截至 2020 年 3 月 31 日 12 时，全球共 202 个国家暴发了新型冠状病毒肺炎疫情。除中国外，其他国家累计确诊 778 465 例，累计治愈 162 717 例，累计死亡 37 185 例（涉及 126 个国家，其中死亡人数前 10 的国家为意大利、西班牙、美国、法国、伊朗、英国、荷兰、德国、比利时、瑞士）。

三、新型冠状病毒肺炎的感染机制

2020 年 1 月 10 日，武汉新型冠状病毒的第一个基因组序列数据被公布，后来陆续有多个从患者身上分离的新型冠状病毒的基因组序列发布。中国科学院上海巴斯德研究所、军事科学院军事医学研究院国家应急防控药物工程技术研究中心及中国科学院分子植物卓越创新中心将武汉新型冠状病毒基因组与 SARS-CoV、MERS-CoV 进行了全基因组比对，发现平均分别有 70% 和 40% 的序列相似性，其中不同冠状病毒与宿主细胞作用的关键 *spike* 基因（编码 S- 蛋白）有更大的差异性（图 1-2-1）。

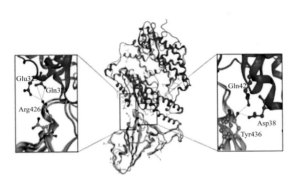

图 1-2-1　新型冠状病毒的预测结构

四、动物源性与新型冠状病毒肺炎

冠状病毒除了本身的特征性变化外，还会随着宿主的转移而变化。随着人类活动范围的不断扩大，一些与人类隔绝的病毒，通过野生动物的传播而感染人类，如 2003 年的 SARS 病毒可能起源于蝙蝠，通过中间宿主果子狸传染给人类。因此，寻找病毒相关的动物源性对了解和控制病毒的传播至关重要。

目前被确诊为新型冠状病毒肺炎的患者，最早出现于武汉。研究人员对 9 例住院患者（其中 8 人曾到过武汉华南海鲜市场）进行病毒分离和基因组测序后发现，该基因组与 2018 年在中国东部舟山发现的 2 种蝙蝠来源的冠状病毒 bat-SL-CoVZC45 和 bat-SL-CoVXC21 序列一致性约为 88%。中国科学院武汉病毒研究所石正丽团队发现 2019-nCoV 与一种蝙蝠的冠状病毒的序列一致性高达 96%。通过对其 7 个保守的非结构蛋白进行对比，发现 nCoV-2019 属于 SARS-CoV，且 2019-nCoV 进入细胞的受体与 SARS-CoV 一样，均为 ACE2。2020 年 2 月，华南农业大学、岭南现代农业科学与技术广东省实验室沈永义教授等科研团队开展的最新研究表明，穿山甲为新型冠状病毒潜在的中间宿主，但截至目前其中间宿主尚无定论。

五、新型冠状病毒肺炎的流行特点

新型冠状病毒主要的传播途径是呼吸道飞沫传播和接触传播，粪-口传播还有待研究，在医疗机构中存在气溶胶传播的可能。病毒输入一个地区后，如不加干预，很容易引起当地聚集性病例的发生，但如果采取严格隔离和增大社交距离等控制措施，可以有效降低发病率。新型冠状病毒几乎人人易感，人类感染后是否具有免疫力还需进一步研究。根据钟南山院士的研究，从确诊和疑似病例上分析，大部分患者分布在 30 ～ 65 岁，其中 56 岁最多，18 岁及以下人群的患病率相对较低（占所有报告病例的 2.4%）；儿童病例多是通过追踪成年患者家庭密切接触者时发现，未发现有儿童传染成年人的情况；确诊和疑似病例年龄分布类似；真正的无症状感染者比例尚不明确，但相对罕见，也不是传播的主要因素。从地域上分析，武汉以外的城市发病年龄更低。每 10 万人中，男性发病率（37%）与女性发病率（27%）具有显著差异（$P < 0.001$），平均潜伏期为 4.75（四分位间距 3.0 ～ 7.2）天。与 SARS-CoV 相比，新型冠状病毒具有更强的传播力和较低的病死率。基于个体层面的监测数据，老年患者的早期发现和治疗十分重要，尤其是老年男性患者。

第三节　新型冠状病毒肺炎的病原学检测价值

根据国家卫健委发布的《新型冠状病毒肺炎诊疗方案（试行第七版）》，将实时荧光逆转录-聚合酶链反应（RT-PCR）和病毒基因组测序作为病原学检测手段。实时荧光 RT-PCR 检测血液中是否存在病毒核酸，诊断有无病原体感染，是最直接有效的方法之一。而 RT-PCR 因其技术灵敏且用途广泛，是核酸检测最常用的技术之一，其原理是将 RNA 的反转录（RT）和 cDNA 的聚合酶链式扩增（PCR）相结合的技术。然而，有些患者临床上表现为新型冠状病毒肺炎，但核酸检测结果却为阴性，这种临床诊断假阴性可能的原因是：①试剂盒的特异性、灵敏度及稳定性有待深入优化与验证，试剂盒质量也有待提升；②采样部位及样本内的病毒含量可能影响检测结果。

目前，最常用的方法为采集鼻咽拭子，然而，鼻咽拭子采集随机性较高，病毒核酸样本的提取可能会受到个体差异的影响。并且，上呼吸道（包括鼻咽部）的病毒量在患者发病的早期可能太少，达不到试剂盒的检出限。另外，样本的保存和运输也很关键。样本可能出现保存不当的现象，这可能会影响病毒核酸的提取率和质量，并影响后续的定量分析。

第四节　新型冠状病毒肺炎的 CT 检测价值

随着对新型冠状病毒肺炎认识的逐步深入，该疾病的特征性 CT 影像改变和动态演变过程更加清晰。由于 CT 分辨率较高，对新型冠状病毒肺炎的诊断敏感性也较高，对于早期诊断、早期隔离、早期治疗及减少传播，进而缩短疫情时间有重要意义。因此，肺部 CT 在新型冠状病毒肺炎的诊断及病情判断方面的作用越来越重要。国家卫健委发布的《新型冠状病毒肺炎诊疗方案（试行第七版）》新型冠状病毒肺炎患者的诊断标准中，新型冠状病毒肺炎 CT 影像学特征是诊断为疑似病例的一个重要条件。

2

第二章

新型冠状病毒肺炎的
表现特点与治疗

第一节　新型冠状病毒肺炎的临床分型

根据国家卫健委发布的《新型冠状病毒肺炎诊疗方案（试行第七版）》，新型冠状病毒肺炎的临床分型可分为轻型、普通型、重型及危重型。

一、轻型

患者临床症状轻微，甚至无临床症状，影像学未见肺炎表现。

二、普通型

患者具有发热、呼吸道等症状，影像学可见肺炎表现。

三、重型

成年患者符合下列任何一条：①出现气促，呼吸频率（respiratory rate，RR）≥ 30 次 / 分；②静息状态下，指血氧饱和度 ≤ 93%；③动脉血氧分压（PaO_2）/ 吸氧浓度（FiO_2）≤ 300 mmHg（1 mmHg=0.133 kPa），高海拔（海拔超过 1000 m）地区应根据公式（PaO_2/FiO_2）×[大气压（mmHg）/760]进行纠正；④肺部影像学显示 24 ~ 48 小时内病灶明显进展 > 50%。

高龄、合并严重基础疾病者易发展为危重型。

四、危重型

成年患者符合下列任何一条：①出现呼吸衰竭，且需要机械通气；②出现休克；③合并其他器官功能衰竭，需 ICU 监护治疗。

第二节　新型冠状病毒肺炎的临床表现

根据目前的流行病学，新型冠状病毒肺炎的潜伏期为 1 ~ 14 天，多为 3 ~ 7 天，但也有报道长达 24 天者。

一、轻型

患者临床仅表现为低热、乏力、干咳等轻度呼吸道症状，有些患者甚至无临床症状，胸部影像学未见肺炎表现。

二、普通型

大多数患者表现为发热、干咳、乏力，少数为咽痛、鼻塞、恶心、腹泻、胸闷、食欲下降、肌肉酸痛、头晕、头痛等，无特异性，胸部影像学可见肺炎表现。

三、重型及危重型

患者发病一周后，一般为 7 ~ 14 天，可出现呼吸困难和/或低氧血症、胸闷、咳嗽、乏力、食欲下降、头晕等较普通型患者更容易出现，此型患者体温可为中低热，甚至无明显发热。严重者可数天甚至数小时内发展为急性呼吸窘迫综合征、脓毒性休克、顽固性代谢性酸中毒、严重凝血功能障碍及多器官功能衰竭。

第三节　新型冠状病毒肺炎的实验室检查

发病早期患者外周血白细胞总数正常或减少，在合并细菌感染时白细胞总数可升高，淋巴细胞绝对值下降，主要为 $CD4^+T$ 细胞和 $CD8^+T$ 细胞的减少。少数患者血小板数量下降，部分患者出现肝酶、肌酐、乳酸脱氢酶、肌酸激酶、凝血酶原降低。多数患者出现 C- 反应蛋白（C-reactive protein，CRP）及红细胞沉降率（erythrocyte sedimentation rate，ESR）升高，降钙素原、肌钙蛋白基本正常。严重患者外周血淋巴细胞进行性下降，D- 二聚体升高。多数重型及危重型患者炎症因子 IL-6、IL-10 升高，但随病情好转可迅速下降。

在鼻咽拭子、痰、肺泡灌洗液、血液、粪便等标本中可检测出新型冠状病毒核酸。咽拭子容易出现假阴性，为提高核酸检测阳性率，我们建议留取痰液标本后尽快送检。

第四节　新型冠状病毒肺炎的诊断标准

一、疑似病例

临床表现：①发热和 / 或呼吸道症状；②新型冠状病毒肺炎典型影像学表现；③早期白细胞总数正常或下降，淋巴细胞计数下降。符合临床表现中的任意两项或三项，且有流行病学史，即可诊断为疑似病例。

二、确诊病例

疑似病例具备以下病原学证据之一：①实时荧光 RT-PCR 检测新型冠状病毒核酸阳性；②病毒基因测序与已知的新型冠状病毒高度同源；③血清新型冠状病毒特异性 IgM 抗体和 IgG 抗体阳性，血清新型冠状病毒特异性 IgG 抗体由阴性或恢复期较急性期 4 倍及以上升高。

第五节　新型冠状病毒肺炎的治疗方案

一、治疗方案

1. 严密监测患者生命体征变化：体温、呼吸节律、频率、深浅及血氧饱和度。

2. 氧疗的患者，根据患者血氧饱和度调整氧流量，必要时及时予经鼻高流量氧疗（high-flow nasal cannula oxygen therapy，HFNCOT）。

3. 使用无创呼吸机辅助通气患者，根据患者潮气量和氧合指数等调整吸气压力、呼气压力及吸氧浓度等参数。

4.气管插管或气管切开患者，需在实施三级防护措施下采用密闭式吸痰，做好人工气道管理。

二、病情观察

1.密切观察患者意识及全身状态，如咳嗽、胸闷、肌肉酸痛、乏力、腹泻、食欲等，注意是否出现症状加重或有新发症状出现。

2.加强患者基础疾病的监测及治疗，如高血压、糖尿病、肾功能不全等。

3.预防并及时处理并发症。

三、药物治疗

（一）轻型

卧床休息，营养支持，保证充分热量。新型冠状病毒肺炎尚缺乏明确有效的抗病毒治疗药物，现阶段可选用 α - 干扰素（成年人每次500 万单位 + 灭菌注射用水 2 mL，雾化吸收，每日 2 次）、洛匹那韦 / 利托那韦（成年人每次 500 mg，每日 2 次）、阿比多尔（成年人每次200 mg，每日 3 次）、磷酸氯喹（成年人 500 mg，每日 2 次）等，需注意抗病毒药物不良反应，如恶心、腹泻等，不建议同时应用 3 种及以上抗病毒药物。

（二）普通型

一般治疗同轻型，严密监测患者症状、体征，如出现持续高热、呼吸困难、血氧饱和度下降等，给予鼻导管吸氧，可试用抗病毒治疗：α - 干扰素（成年人每次 500 万单位 + 灭菌注射用水 2 mL，雾化吸收，每日 2 次）、洛匹那韦 / 利托那韦（成年人每次 500 mg，每日 2 次）、阿比多尔（成年人每次 200 mg，每日 3 次）、磷酸氯喹（成年人 500 mg，每日 2 次）等。当氧合指数＜ 300 时立即参照重型标准执行。

（三）重型

治疗原则：在对症治疗的基础上，积极治疗并发症，治疗基础疾病，预防继发感染，及时进行器官功能支持，必要时经鼻高流量吸氧、无创呼吸机通气，不推荐对 HFNCOT 治疗失败的患者常规使用无创正压通气。我们有如下建议。

1. 持续监测血氧饱和度、血气分析，定期复查胸部 CT。

2. 抗病毒治疗：可选用 α- 干扰素（成年人每次 500 万单位 + 灭菌注射用水 2 mL，雾化吸收，每日 2 次）、洛匹那韦 / 利托那韦（成年人 500 mg，每日 2 次）、阿比多尔（成年人 200 mg，每日 3 次）、磷酸氯喹（成年人 500 mg，每日 2 次）等。

3. 早期诊断为重型时立即给予小剂量糖皮质激素治疗［甲泼尼龙 0.5 ~ 1 mg/（kg·d），根据症状、血氧饱和度改善情况逐步减量至停用，疗程为 3 ~ 10 天］。

4. 可联用人免疫球蛋白。

5. 不推荐常规预防性使用抗菌药物，有感染征象（如白细胞升高等），静脉用抗菌素。

6. 调节肠道微生态及其他支持治疗。

（四）危重型

有创机械通气：实行小潮气量（4 ~ 6 mL/kg）和低吸气压力（平台压 < 30 cmH$_2$O）等肺保护性机械通气策略，根据急性呼吸窘迫综合征（acute respiratory distress syndrome，ARDS）严重程度设置呼气末正压通气（positive end expiratory pressure，PEEP），以减少呼吸机相关肺损伤，可行肺复张治疗，俯卧位通气，必要时可考虑体外膜肺氧合（extracorporeal membrane oxygenation，ECMO）治疗。我们有如下建议。

1. 密切监测血气分析、床边胸片。

2. 甲泼尼龙 80 ~ 160 mg/d，根据患者症状、氧饱和度改善情况逐步减量至停用。

3. 抗病毒治疗：可选用 α - 干扰素（成年人每次 500 万单位 + 灭菌注射用水 2 mL， 雾化吸收，每日 2 次）、洛匹那韦 / 利托那韦（成年人每次 500 mg，每日 2 次）、阿比多尔（成年人每次 200 mg，每日 3 次）、磷酸氯喹（成年人 500 mg，每日 2 次）等。

4. 可联用人免疫球蛋白。

5. 有感染征象（如白细胞升高等），静脉用抗菌素。

6. 调节肠道微生态及其他支持治疗。

7. 人工肝治疗。

8. 康复者血浆治疗。

9. 免疫治疗，对于 IL-6 水平升高者，可试用托珠单抗治疗。

10. 合并休克治疗：①液体复苏：可选择生理盐水、平衡液，必要时可予人血白蛋白补充；②血管活性药物：推荐去甲肾上腺素作为首选血管活性药物，其他可选择多巴胺、垂体后叶素等。

四、心理评估及支持

1. 评估患者的认知改变、情绪反应和行为变化，给予患者心理调适等干预措施。

2. 提供恰当的情感支持，鼓励患者树立战胜疾病的信心。

3. 提供连续的正确的信息支持，消除不确定感和焦虑情绪。

4. 做好患者的健康指导，保证充足的睡眠及良好的心理状态。

五、营养支持

1. 加强营养支持，给予高热量、高蛋白、高维生素、易消化饮食。

2. 重症患者给予肠内或肠外营养支持，能量供应 25 ~ 35 kcal/(kg·d)，尽早启动肠内营养，预防反流误吸。

六、呼吸康复锻炼

选择合适的呼吸康复锻炼方式，如气道廓清训练、呼吸操、缩唇呼吸、腹式呼吸等。

七、中医辨证施治

新型冠状病毒肺炎可分为初期、中期、重症期及恢复期。初期分寒湿郁肺与外寒内热，中期为寒热错杂，重症期为疫毒内闭，恢复期为肺脾气虚。根据分期、分型辨证论治，寒热并用法始终贯穿其中。

第六节　新型冠状病毒肺炎患者的出院标准与随访

体温恢复正常 3 天以上，呼吸道症状明显好转，肺内病灶明显吸收，连续 2 次呼吸道病原核酸检测阴性（采样间隔至少 1 天）。鉴于近期发现粪内能检测到核酸阳性，所以我们将粪病原核酸检测阴性纳入出院标准。

出院后，居家隔离 14 天，2 周、1 个月、3 个月、6 个月、1 年门诊随访，复诊时重点复查血常规、血生化、血氧饱和度、肺部 CT、肺功能，必要时进行新型冠状病毒病原学检测。

3

第三章

新型冠状病毒肺炎的
检查流程与诊断规范

新型冠状病毒肺炎疫情防控形势严峻，影像学检查作为诊断新型冠状病毒肺炎的重要环节，在新型冠状病毒肺炎的筛查、诊断、病情预测与预后等方面发挥着重要作用。目前，肺部 CT 作为早期诊断的重要检查手段，放射技师位于疫情防控第一线，面临感染防控和放射防护的双重责任与压力，规范影像学检查流程显得尤为重要。本流程参照国家卫健委印发的《新型冠状病毒肺炎防控方案（第六版）》、中华医学会影像技术分会发布的《新型冠状病毒（2019-nCoV）感染肺炎放射检查方案与感染防控专家共识（第一版）》，结合实际工作经验，制定了不同影像学检查设备及根据不同患者身体状况的分类检查流程。

第一节　新型冠状病毒肺炎患者的检查流程

为了更好地进行疫情防控，防止交叉感染，尽量创造条件设立独立的医学影像检查区域或专用放射检查设备，固定专人进行发热患者的影像学检查工作。

一、专区与专机

要严格划分污染区、潜在污染区与清洁区，严格按照防控要求，在各自相应区域内工作，不得违规穿越或混淆分区界限造成污染。我们提倡有条件的医院设立单独的 CT 机房与数字化 X 线摄影（digital radiography，DR）机房，并且配有独立的候诊区域用于接诊上述发热患者。在机房选择上，应选择具有独立操作间的机房，不得与其他机器共用操作间；若无法达到上述条件，检查后对于机房内及操作间的消毒工作应严格按照消毒流程进行操作，并且把与操作间相连接的其他机房进行空气消毒。普通患者将在划定的区域就诊，减小与疑似、确诊新型冠状病毒肺炎患者接触的可能性，减小院内感染或医源性感染的概率。

二、专人

科内合理安排人员，须固定专人分班进行上述发热患者的接诊工作，需在医院专门的隔离区域内工作和生活，一个工作周期结束后进入专用隔离区进行医学观察，观察期结束后检测核酸及肺部 CT，检查无异常则可恢复正常生活，重返工作岗位。直接与发热、疑似和确诊新型冠状病毒肺炎患者发生近距离接触者，存在较大的职业暴露风险，要注意隔离与防护，最大限度地减小医务人员院内感染的风险。医务人员进入发热专用机房必须按二级防护标准准备：工作服外加一次性隔离衣或防护服、N95 口罩、护目镜或一次性护目屏、一次性帽子、单层乳胶手套。其余机房医务人员应严格执行一级防护。同时，科内要强调手卫生的重要性，医务人员要自觉落实好手卫生的工作，保护患者，也保护自己。

三、放射诊断检查中的感染防控等级

（一）一般防护

一般防护适用于放射诊断室、后处理室、信息管理室等远离患者的工作人员。戴一次性工作帽、一次性医用外科口罩，穿工作服，注意手卫生。

（二）一级防护

一级防护适用于非发热患者的预检分诊、登记处、取片处、普通放射检查室等区域的工作人员。戴一次性工作帽、一次性医用外科口罩（接触有流行病学史患者时用 N95 型或以上等级医用防护口罩），穿工作服（接触有流行病学史患者时加穿隔离衣），必要时戴一次性乳胶手套，严格执行手卫生。

（三）二级防护

二级防护适用于发热门诊、感染门诊、呼吸门诊、隔离病房、专用

放射检查室等场所对疑似和确诊新型冠状病毒肺炎患者进行放射检查的近距离操作人员。戴一次性工作帽、N95 型或以上等级医用防护口罩、护目镜或防护面屏、一次性乳胶手套，穿医用防护服（在隔离病房时加穿隔离衣）、一次性鞋套或靴套，严格执行手卫生。

（四）三级防护

三级防护适用于在相对封闭的环境中并长时间暴露于高浓度气溶胶的情况下，为疑似或确诊重症新型冠状病毒肺炎患者进行放射检查的近距离操作人员。在二级防护基础上，加戴防护面屏、护目镜、全面型呼吸防护器或正压式头套，严格执行手卫生。

感染防控等级的确定，应以所接触的患者类型、与患者接触的暴露风险程度为依据，而不应仅限定于以上提及的具体场所。

（五）防护服穿脱

1. 穿防护用品流程：七步洗手→戴帽子→戴医用防护口罩（N95，漏气试验）→穿防护服（脱鞋后）→戴乳胶手套（内层）→穿一次性隔离衣→戴乳胶手套（外层）→穿胶靴→穿靴套→戴护目镜或防护面屏→检查穿戴严密性。

2. 脱防护用品流程

（1）污染区：清除可见污物→手卫生→脱外层鞋套→手卫生→脱隔离衣连同外层手套→手卫生。

（2）半污染区：摘护目镜或防护面屏→手卫生→脱防护服连同内层手套和靴套→手卫生—摘医用防护口罩（N95）→摘帽子→七步洗手。

（六）放射科机房终末消毒标准

1. 擦拭消毒所有接触过的设备及物品表面，消毒液可采用 75% 酒精或 1000 mg/L 含氯消毒液，30 分钟后再用清水擦拭。

2.空气消毒：可使用循环空气消毒机持续消毒，或者无人状态下持续使用紫外线照射消毒，每次 30 分钟。

3.地面用 500 mg/L 含氯消毒液清洁，30 分钟后用清水清洁。

4.所有垃圾袋以鹅颈法结扎后放指定区域。患者所有的废弃物应当视为感染性医疗废物，严格依照《医疗废物管理条例》和《医疗卫生机构医疗废物管理办法》处理。

第二节 发热患者（有流行病学史）、疑似及确诊新型冠状病毒肺炎患者的检查流程

一、技师检查前准备

为了最大限度地保护科内医护人员，我们建议将 DR 与 CT 检查都由同一技师进行操作。操作前，技师应严格执行二级防护，如果遇到吸痰、呼吸道采样、气管插管及气管切开等有可能发生患者呼吸道分泌物、体内物质的喷射或飞溅的情况时，必须执行三级防护。

二、患者检查前准备

患者检查前应由当班护士提前与放射科取得联系，并告知患者情况，等待放射科人员打开患者专用通道入口大门。患者检查全程戴医用外科口罩或 N95 口罩，根据检查部位，提前除去该部位的金属饰物和其他高密度物品（如项链、耳环、有金属拉链的衣物等）。可以自主活动的患者，在护士进行宣教工作后，陪同前往检查室进行检查。需推车或推床运送的患者，护士在进行严格的手消毒后，护送患者至检查室进行检查。保卫科人员应协同护送，疏散就诊人员，并劝导就诊人员保持 1.5 m 以上的距离，走专用通道，应尽可能避免接触周围环境与行人，在患者结束检查后，运送回隔离区，并对运送工具及时进行消毒。

三、检查过程及要求

检查前,技师应认真核对申请单及注意事项,明确检查目的和要求,询问患者姓名,核对住院患者腕带,做好"三查七对"工作,做好非检查部位的辐射防护,并按要求进行呼吸训练。尽量避免与患者的近距离交流,除了摆位以外,在保障患者安全的前提下,应与患者保持 1 ~ 1.5 m 或以上的距离。有条件的医院应尽可能利用机器的智能升降床系统进行检查。

因病情需要注射对比剂进行检查或者其他需要护士直接接触患者的情况时,护士应按要求执行二级防护。

四、检查结束后的消毒工作

在患者检查结束后,更换床单,擦拭消毒所有接触过的设备及物品表面。若为疑似或确诊新型冠状病毒肺炎患者,应立即用空气消毒机进行空气消毒 30 分钟,同时配置 1000 mg/L 含氯消毒液拖地,后用清水再次清洁地面。将污染的一次性用物放入双层医疗垃圾袋,并采用鹅颈式密闭扎口后用含氯消毒液或 75% 酒精喷射垃圾袋外表面,再套一个黄色垃圾袋,进行鹅颈式包扎后,贴"新型冠状病毒肺炎"标签,联系保洁办,由专人密封转运医疗废物。机房内用 1000 mg/L 的含氯消毒液浸泡的毛巾擦拭桌面、门及门把手等所有物品,根据发生污染的可能性由低到高依次擦拭。所有流程结束后,按七步洗手法,严格执行手卫生。

(注意:在疑似与确诊新型冠状病毒肺炎患者同时就诊时,应先做疑似患者,再做确诊患者,同时,在两名患者之间要严格执行上述消毒工作。)

第三节 普通发热患者、普通患者(检查中发现疑似新型冠状病毒肺炎患者)的检查流程

一、技师检查前准备

操作前,技师应严格执行一级防护,如果遇到吸痰、呼吸道采样、气管插管及气管切开等有可能发生患者呼吸道分泌物、体内物质的喷射或飞溅的情况时,必须执行二级防护。

二、患者检查前准备

患者检查过程中,在不影响图像质量的前提下,应全程戴医用外科口罩或 N95 口罩。根据检查部位,除去该部位的金属饰物和其他高密度物品(如项链、耳环、有金属拉链的衣物等)。

三、检查过程及要求

检查前,技师应认真核对申请单及注意事项,明确检查目的和要求,询问患者姓名,核对住院患者腕带,做好"三查七对"工作。做好非检查部位的辐射防护,并按要求进行呼吸训练。

四、检查方法

检查后,应仔细浏览图像,评估是否有疑似新型冠状病毒肺炎可能。若有疑似倾向,立刻联系诊断组医师协助诊断,同时,请患者在机房内等候进行隔离,技师更换个人防护用品。如诊断医师也高度怀疑,向现场领导或高年资医师汇报,并电话通知发热门诊,由专人护送患者离开检查室。将机房门口其余等候的患者,做好分流工作。

五、检查结束后的消毒工作

在患者检查结束后,更换床单,擦拭消毒所有接触过的设备及物品表面。若为疑似患者,应立即用空气消毒机进行空气消毒 30 分钟,同

时配置 500 mg/L 含氯消毒液拖地，后用清水再次清洁地面。将污染的一次性用物放入双层医疗垃圾袋，并采用鹅颈式密闭扎口后用含氯消毒液或 75% 酒精喷射垃圾袋外表面，再套一个黄色垃圾袋，进行鹅颈式包扎后，贴"新型冠状病毒肺炎"标签，联系保洁办，由专人密封转运医疗废物。机房内用 1000 mg/L 的含氯消毒液浸泡的毛巾擦拭桌面、门及门把手等所有物品。所有流程结束后，按七步洗手法，严格执行手卫生。管理好进出机房的每一个入口，不允许无关人员入内。

第四节　普通发热患者、普通患者的检查流程

一、技师检查前准备

操作前，技师应严格执行一级防护，如果遇到需吸痰、呼吸道采样、气管插管及气管切开等有可能发生患者呼吸道分泌物、体内物质的喷射或飞溅的情况时，必须执行二级防护（图 3-4-1）。

二、患者检查前准备

患者检查过程中，在不影响图像质量的前提下，应全程戴医用外科口罩或 N95 口罩。根据检查部位，除去该部位的金属饰物和其他高密度物品（如项链、耳环、有金属拉链的衣物等）。

三、检查过程及要求

检查前，技师应认真核对申请单及注意事项，明确检查目的和要求，询问患者姓名，核对住院患者腕带，做好"三查七对"工作。做好非检查部位的辐射防护，并按要求进行呼吸训练。

四、检查结束后的消毒工作

普通发热患者同急诊患者同等对待，30 分钟内出具报告。普通机

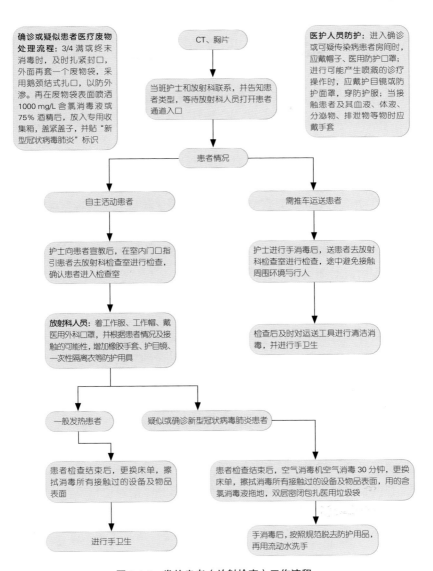

图 3-4-1　发热患者（放射检查）工作流程

房应执行每日 2 次的消毒工作，对机房物品及设备表面用可达高水平消毒的湿巾进行擦拭，当班人员上、下午下班前各对自己工作区域设备进行一次常规消毒。

第五节　发热患者（有流行病学史）、疑似及确诊新型冠状病毒肺炎患者床旁操作的检查流程

一、技师检查前准备

医院应准备一台移动 DR 作为专门设备放在隔离病房专供发热患者（有流行病学史）、疑似新型冠状病毒及确诊新型冠状病毒患者使用。操作前，技师应严格执行二级防护，如果遇到吸痰、呼吸道采样、气管插管及气管切开等有可能发生患者呼吸道分泌物、体内物质的喷射或飞溅的情况时，必须执行三级防护。

二、患者检查前准备

患者检查过程中，在不影响图像质量的前提下，应全程戴医用外科口罩或 N95 口罩。根据检查部位，除去该部位的金属饰物和其他高密度物品（如项链、耳环、有金属拉链的衣物等）。

三、检查过程及要求

检查前，技师应认真核对申请单及注意事项，明确检查目的和要求，询问患者姓名，核对住院患者腕带，做好"三查七对"工作。做好非检查部位的辐射防护，并按要求进行呼吸训练。尽量避免与患者的近距离交流，除了摆位以外，在保障患者安全的前提下，应与患者保持 1 ~ 1.5 m 或以上的距离。

四、检查结束后的消毒工作

在患者检查结束后，擦拭消毒所有接触过的设备及物品表面。按七步洗手法，严格执行手卫生。拍摄技师作为密切接触者，在隔离区内待命工作 2 周，出隔离病房后进行医学观察，观察期结束后检测核酸及肺部 CT 无异常则可恢复正常工作和生活。

第六节 新型冠状病毒肺炎的检查技术

一、DR 检查方案

（一）检查注意事项

1. 配置一台专用 DR 作为新型冠状病毒肺炎患者专用机。

2. 严格按照上述的消毒措施进行设备和机房管理。

3. 危重患者建议床旁摄片。

（二）成年人放射检查方案

1. 摄影距离：180 cm。

2. 滤线栅：栅比最低 10：1。

3. 曝光条件：125 kV，电离室自动曝光技术。

4. 摄影体位：后前位，中心线对准第六胸椎水平处垂直于探测器入射。

5. 防护要求：使用铅围裙等尽可能遮挡身体其他部位。

6. 呼吸要求：深吸气末屏气采集。

（三）0 ~ 3 岁和 3 岁以上不合作者放射检查方案

1. 摄影距离：100 cm。

2. 滤线栅：不使用。

3. 曝光条件：50 ～ 60 kV，0.6 ～ 2 mAs。

4. 摄影体位：前后位，需患者家属帮助固定体位，中心线对准两乳头连线的中心垂直射入。

5. 防护要求：使用铅围裙等尽可能遮挡身体其他部位。

（四）移动床旁 X 线摄影检查方案

1. 在新型冠状病毒肺炎隔离病区等重点区域配备专用移动床旁 X 线机，专门为危重患者拍摄。

2. 技师进新型冠状病毒肺炎隔离病区前应严格执行二级防护，若遇到如吸痰、呼吸道采样、气管插管及气管切开等有可能发生患者呼吸道分泌物、体内物质的喷射或飞溅的工作时，必须执行三级防护。

3. 床旁拍摄，做好平板探测器或者 IP 板的防护，建议用塑料袋套上平板，使用后进行消毒处理。

二、CT 检查方案

（一）检查注意事项

1. 指定 CT、指定人员对发热患者进行检查，机房应选择独立操作间，不与其他机器共用操作间，候诊厅亦为独立空间。

2. 对确诊新型冠状病毒患者，在院内感染部门、医务室、放射科、病房多点协调下，设立患者"运送→检查→返回病区"的检查闭环流程及路径。

3. 发热门诊患者从指定通道进入 CT 机房，检查完成后原路返回发热门诊。

4. 确诊患者扫描完成后，按放射科机房终末消毒标准进行机房消毒。

5. CT 操作技师在检查完成后，执行手卫生。

6.机房采用新风系统中央空调的,将空调送风量和排风量开到最大;机房采用普通中央空调的,应关闭机房、操作间中央空调,开启备用独立空调,如果没有独立空调,做完检查消毒后再开启中央空调。

7.检查床应铺一次性中单,避免折叠,覆盖整个检查床面;防护用品使用时要用一次性中单与患者身体、衣物相隔离。

检查中注意"三查七对",明确检查目的和要求;患者检查应全程戴医用外科口罩或 N95 医用防护口罩(包括患者和陪护人员);去除检查区域高密度物品。扫描前对患者进行呼吸训练,一般采用吸气末屏气,呼吸不能配合的患者嘱其平静呼吸,避免咳嗽。

检查技师在交代检查注意事项时尽量采用对讲方式。对于能够配合的患者, 检查技师在保证患者安全的前提下,可在操作室声控引导患者摆位,亦可请陪同人员协助患者上检查床;需要检查技师亲自摆位时,尽量与患者保持 1 m 以上距离,如无法保证 1 m 以上距离,头尽量远离患者呼吸道。接触患者前后及时用速干手消毒液洗手;就检患者进入检查区域和整个检查过程中必须佩戴口罩。

(二)CT 扫描方案

1.扫描体位:常规取仰卧位,两臂上举抱头。手臂上举困难者,可置于身体两侧。

2.扫描方式:螺旋扫描。

3.扫描范围:从肺尖扫描至膈底(包括双侧肋膈角),对憋气不佳的患者从膈底扫描至肺尖(肺底部呼吸运动幅度大于肺尖部),减少双肺下野因屏气不佳造成的呼吸运动伪影,保证图像质量。

4.扫描参数:一般采用螺旋扫描(120 kV),使用智能辐射剂量跟踪技术(50 ~ 350 mAs),采集层厚 0.5 ~ 1.5 mm。

5.儿童应采用低剂量扫描,辐射剂量可低至 20 mAs。

（三）CT 图像重建

1. 常规图像重建：常规以 5 mm 层厚分别重建出肺窗图像（肺窗：窗宽 1000 ~ 1500 Hu，窗位 -650 ~ -500 Hu）和纵隔窗图像（纵隔窗：窗宽 250 ~ 300 Hu，窗位 30 ~ 50 Hu）。

2. 薄层图像重建：常规以 1 mm 以下层厚重建出薄层肺窗图像（肺窗：窗宽 1000 ~ 1500 Hu，窗位 -650 ~ -500 Hu）。

第七节　新型冠状病毒肺炎的诊断规范

一、适用对象

时有不明原因的发热（体温＞37.3℃）或不明原因的急性呼吸道感染的患者，如有武汉旅居接触史、本地确诊或疑似患者接触史，作为重点筛查人群。

二、检查方式

DR 或 CT 检查，首选 CT 检查。

三、影像结果确认

（一）CT 检查（首选）或 DR 检查无异常

执行常规报告，建议临床相关检查，14 天后复查仍无异常，则排除诊断。

（二）CT 检查（首选）或 DR 检查发现异常

肺部 CT 或 DR 出现单发或多发小斑片状影、磨玻璃影伴或不伴有间质性改变，以双肺中下肺野、外带为著，进展期双肺多发磨玻璃影及浸润影，严重者出现肺实变。

1. 对出现上述典型影像表现的患者，医师审核，并上报危急值，如果影像学确诊，建议临床做相关实验室检查，最终明确诊断。

2. 对影像表现不典型的患者，如果当班医师仍首选考虑疑似新型冠状病毒肺炎，给予疑似诊断，审核并上报危急值，同时建议临床完善相关检查。

3. 对影像表现不典型患者，如果当班医师不能确定，请胸组组长或副组长会诊，仍不能诊断时请示科主任，如果认为疑似诊断，按上述 2 条款执行；如果认为排除诊断，按 1 条款执行（图 3-7-1）。

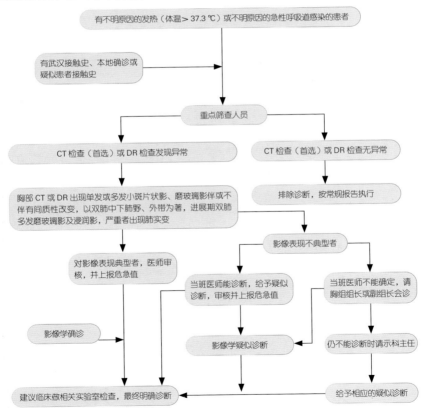

图 3-7-1　放射科关于新型冠状病毒肺炎的诊断流程

4

第四章

新型冠状病毒肺炎的影像分期与病理基础

第一节　新型冠状病毒肺炎的影像分期

目前尚缺乏系统的放射学表现与病例对照研究资料。基于目前的临床实践，根据病变受累的范围和表现，推荐将新型冠状病毒肺炎的 CT 表现分为 4 个阶段：早期、进展期、重症期及消散期。

一、早期

1.病变分布：多分布于中、下叶，多位于胸膜下或叶间裂下，或者沿支气管血管束分布。

2.病灶数目：常为双肺多发。

3.病灶密度：①肺内多见磨玻璃密度影，细支气管管壁有增厚，血管影增粗，边缘欠光整，邻近的叶间胸膜有轻度增厚；②肺实变范围小，可见细支气管的空气支气管征；③病灶密度不均匀；④磨玻璃密度影可单独存在，也可与实变同时存在。

4.病灶形态：不规则或扇形多见，也可见片状或类圆形，一般不累及肺段。

5.其他肺外表现：无基础疾病患者，无纵隔淋巴结肿大，无胸腔积液。

二、进展期

1.病灶分布：分布区域增多、增大，以胸膜下为主，可累及多个肺叶。

2.病灶形态：呈不规则形、扇形或楔形。

3.病灶数目：双肺多发。

4.病变范围：范围增大，常见有多发新病灶出现，呈散在多灶性、斑片状甚至弥漫状，可融合成大片，双侧非对称性。原有磨玻璃密度影或实变影也可融合或部分吸收，融合后病变范围和形态常发生变化，不完全沿支气管血管束分布。

5.肺外表现：少部分出现胸腔积液或纵隔淋巴结肿大。

三、重症期

1.病变进一步进展，双肺弥漫性实变，密度不均，其内有空气支气管征和支气管扩张；非实变区可呈斑片状磨玻璃密度影，双肺大部分受累时呈"白肺"表现。48小时病灶范围增加50%，以实变为主，合并磨玻璃密度影，空气支气管征，多发条索影。

2.肺外表现：叶间胸膜和双侧胸膜常见增厚，并有少量胸腔积液，呈游离消散或局部包裹表现。

四、消散期

1.多见于发病后1周左右，病变范围缩小，密度降低，肺实变逐渐消失，渗出物吸收或机化，病灶可完全吸收、部分残留条索影。

2.影像上疾病改善的表现一般晚于临床症状，部分病灶范围增大，或出现新的病灶。

第二节　新型冠状病毒肺炎的病理基础

一、新型冠状病毒的病原学特点

新型冠状病毒属于β属，有包膜，病毒颗粒呈圆形或椭圆形，常为多形性，直径为60～140 nm，其基因特征与急性呼吸窘迫综合征相关的冠状病毒（SARS-CoV）和中东呼吸综合征相关的冠状病毒（MERS-CoV）有明显区别。目前研究显示与蝙蝠SARS样冠状病毒（bat-SL-CoVZC45）同源性达85%以上。在体外分离培养时，2019-nCoV在96小时左右即可在人呼吸道上皮细胞内发现，而在Vero E6和Huh-7细胞系中分离培养约需6天（图4-2-1）。

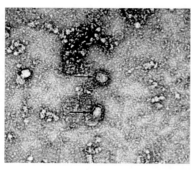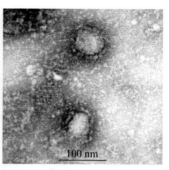

图 4-2-1　新型冠状病毒（↑）电镜图

（图片来源：https://new.qq.com/omn/20200124/20200124A0AXVQ00.html）

二、新型冠状病毒肺炎的解剖组织病理

　　有研究表明：组织学检查显示双侧弥漫性肺泡损伤，伴细胞纤维黏液性渗出（图 4-2-2）；右肺组织出现明显的肺泡上皮脱落和肺透明膜形成，提示 ARDS（图 4-2-2A），左肺组织表现为肺水肿和肺透明膜形成，提示早期 ARDS（图 4-2-2B），双肺中均可见间质内以淋巴细胞为主的单个核细胞炎性浸润；在肺泡腔中出现多核巨细胞和非典型增大的肺泡细胞，其中非典型增大的肺泡细胞具有较大的细胞核、双嗜性的细胞质内颗粒和明显的核仁，表现出病毒性细胞病变样改变（viral cytopathic-like changes）；未发现明显核内或胞浆内病毒包涵体；COVID-19 的病理特征与 SARS 和 MERS 冠状病毒感染的病理特征非常相似。

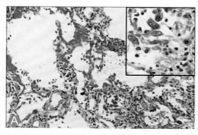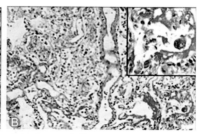

图 4-2-2　一个重症新型冠状病毒肺炎患者的右肺（A）和左肺（B）的病理学表现

（HE 染色，×10）

三、新型冠状病毒肺炎的影像病理特点

次级肺小叶是肺的基本结构单位，呈多边形，有结缔组织包绕，内有肺泡，主要包括小叶核心、小叶周边、小叶间隔及小叶实质。

小叶核心主要包括细支气管和伴行肺动脉，其次为淋巴管，周围由间质包绕（为结缔组织鞘）。

小叶周边走行于小叶交界处（位于小叶周边），内容同小叶核心，为其他小叶之小叶核心，主要包括细支气管和伴行小动脉，其次为淋巴管，由间质包绕（为结缔组织鞘）。

小叶间隔结缔组织板，包绕分割肺小叶，主要包括静脉和淋巴管。

小叶实质主要为肺泡（图 4-2-3）。

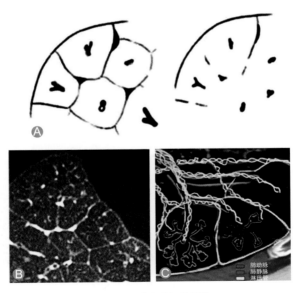

图 4-2-3　肺小叶相关图片

A. 正常肺小叶示意图；B. 肺小叶高分辨率 CT 图；C. 肺小叶间隔示意图

空气支气管征：病原侵犯上皮细胞，造成支气管壁炎性增厚、肿胀，但不阻塞细支气管（图 4-2-4A）。

肺内磨玻璃密度影：病原侵犯细支气管和肺泡上皮，并于上皮细胞内复制，引发非血性渗出。该渗出含受累上皮细胞、淋巴细胞等炎性细胞，与蛋白、纤维素等形成膜性物，该膜半稀半稠，比一般细菌初期稠，比肺泡出血稀。病理：气腔部分填充，肺泡间质增厚或小叶间隔轻度增厚，肺泡部分塌陷，毛细血管血容量增加（图 4-2-4B，图 4-2-4C）。

实变：气腔完全充填（图 4-2-4D，图 4-2-4E）。

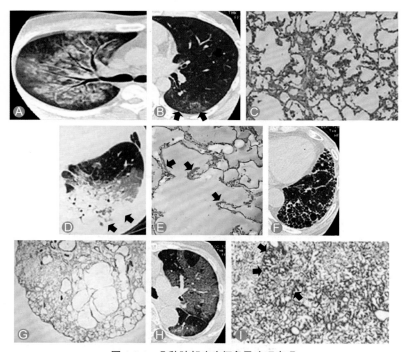

图 4-2-4　几种肺部疾病征象及病理表现

A. 空气支气管征表现；B. 左肺胸膜下磨玻璃密度影 （↑）；C. 左肺胸膜下磨玻璃密度影的病理表现（HE 染色，×10）；D. 左肺实变影 （↑）E. 左肺实变影的病理表现（HE 染色，×100）；F. 左肺"蜂窝征"；G. 左肺"蜂窝征"的病理表现（HE 染色，×10）；H. 左肺"碎石路征" （↑）；I. 左肺"碎石路征"的病理表现（HE 染色，×10）

"蜂窝征"：气囊聚合，代表纤维化。病理：牵拉型支气管扩张的横切，周围纤维化牵拉导致气腔扩张（图 4-2-4F，图 4-2-4G）。

"碎石路征"：磨玻璃影伴下叶内网，代表间质和气腔均可被累及（图 4-2-4H，图 4-2-4I）。

第三节 新型冠状病毒肺炎的临床与病理改变

有研究表明：病毒侵入人体后，一方面由于侵入细胞，导致人体内组织器官受损，引起相应的功能损伤；另一方面人体的免疫细胞会释放出各种细胞因子和自由基等物质对侵入的病毒进行攻击，从而导致器官损害，尤其是过度的免疫反应会导致机体组织器官严重损伤。各种病毒引起的病毒性肺炎虽然可有各种表现，但一般表现为几种可能的肺损伤改变，包括弥漫性肺泡损伤、急性支气管炎、机化性肺炎和弥漫性间质性肺炎等。

早期阶段：病毒进入气道内上皮细胞刺激呼吸道引起反射性咳嗽，但尚未引起肺泡的渗出性炎，仅仅表现为急性间质性炎，以少、中等量淋巴细胞为主的肺泡间隔炎细胞浸润，患者临床表现为发热、干咳等症状。

急性渗出期：组织学上表现为弥漫性肺泡上皮损伤、区域性肺水肿及部分肺泡腔内透明膜形成，感染的肺泡上皮内可能会见到病毒包涵体，临床上患者可有呼吸憋闷、咳痰等症状，影像学检查可有多发小斑片状影（图 4-3-1A，图 4-3-1B）。

脱屑变期：固有或增生的肺泡上皮、终末细支气管上皮及基底膜解离，脱落入肺泡腔内，部分上皮细胞坏死或凋亡，并与炎性渗出物混杂，导致肺泡腔完全被炎性渗出和坏死物填满（图 4-3-1C，图 4-3-1D）。此时，患者会出现明显的呼吸困难，甚至出现 ARDS，引起一系列的体内酸碱失衡和电解质失调，尤其对于有基础疾病的中老年患者，往往因呼吸、循环功能等衰竭而死亡；影像学表现为"白肺征"。

修复期：如果经过积极治疗或提高患者自身的抵抗力增加，病变会转变为增生修复期，表现为肺泡上皮及终末细支气管上皮的增生，早期纤维化和肺泡腔肾小球样机化等。

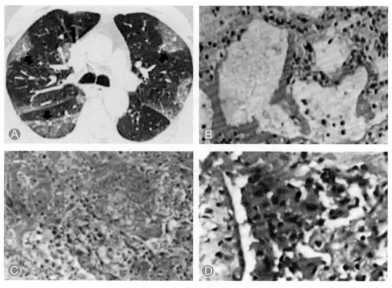

图 4-3-1　新型冠状病毒肺炎肺部 CT 及病理改变

A. 双肺多发性磨片阴影（ ➡ ）；B. 肺泡腔内透明膜形成（HE 染色，×100）；C. 肺泡腔内出血及渗出（HE 染色，×10）；D. 肺泡腔内增生及脱落的上皮细胞团（HE 染色，×20）

5

第五章

新型冠状病毒肺炎早期肺部 CT 表现特点

新型冠状病毒肺炎早期病灶多位于肺外周或胸膜下，双肺下叶为主；常为双肺多发病灶，单发少见；病灶以不规则形、扇形多见，也可见片状或类圆形，病灶一般不累及整个肺段；病灶密度不均匀，以磨玻璃密度影多见，其内可见增粗血管及支气管穿行，伴或不伴有小叶间隔网格状增厚。轻症者病灶多以磨玻璃密度影单独存在，重症者可合并实变，或以实变为主，其内可见空气支气管征；病灶长轴平行于胸膜。无肺部其他疾病者，一般无纵隔和肺门淋巴结肿大，未见胸膜增厚或胸腔积液。

第一节 新型冠状病毒肺炎早期轻症 CT 表现特点

一、病灶分布、形态及数目

常为双肺多发病灶，位于肺外周带或胸膜下，以双肺下叶多见；病灶以不规则形及扇形多见（图 5-1-1）。

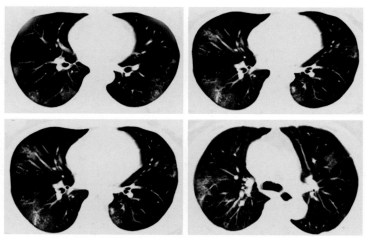

图 5-1-1 双肺叶胸膜下见多发斑片状、扇形磨玻璃高密度影，边界不清

二、磨玻璃密度影

肺内密度增高的模糊影，其内可见高密度肺血管影，提示肺泡腔内渗液、肺泡壁肿胀或肺泡间隔炎症。肺内磨玻璃病灶内可合并增粗血管、小叶间隔增厚或空气支气管征（图 5-1-2）。

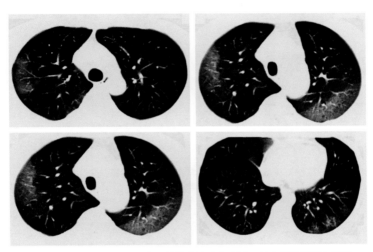

图 5-1-2 双肺叶胸膜下分布斑片状磨玻璃密度影，其内可见增粗血管影

三、"碎石路征"

高分辨率 CT 可见小叶间隔增厚和小叶内间隔线影叠加在磨玻璃不透明的背景上，形状类似不规则的铺路石（图 5-1-3）。

四、空气支气管征

实变的肺组织内含气的支气管呈树枝状低密度影（图 5-1-4）。

五、增粗血管影

磨玻璃密度影内或周围可见增粗的血管影（图 5-1-5）。

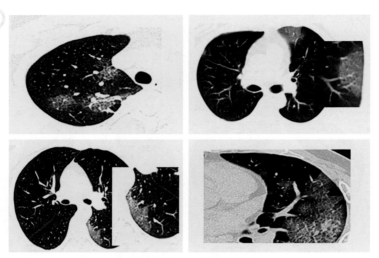

图 5-1-3　双肺叶见磨玻璃斑片影，其内小叶间隔增厚，呈"碎石路征"，
并可见增粗血管影

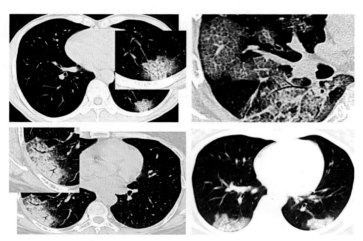

图 5-1-4　双肺叶见斑片状磨玻璃高密度影，其内可见空气支气管征，部
分可见"碎石路征"及增粗血管影

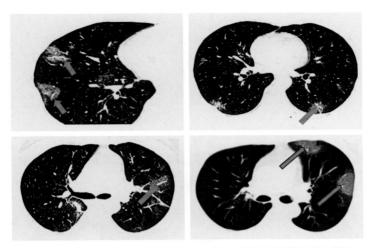

图 5-1-5　双肺叶见磨玻璃斑片影（⬆），其内或周围可见增粗的血管影

六、胸膜下线

病灶长轴与胸膜平行，提示病变首先累及皮层肺组织（图 5-1-6）。

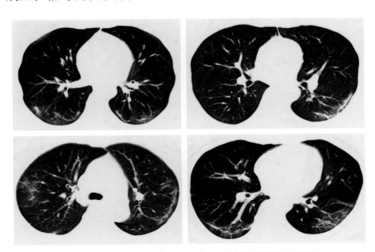

图 5-1-6　双肺叶胸膜下见平行于胸膜的弧形高密度影

七、其他

无肺部其他疾病者，一般无肺门、纵隔淋巴结肿大或胸腔积液。

第二节　新型冠状病毒肺炎早期重症 CT 表现特点

新型冠状病毒肺炎早期重症病灶范围较轻症广，以磨玻璃密度影和实变影为主，仍以胸膜下常见。磨玻璃密度影病灶内常可见增粗血管及"碎石路征"，亦可见空气支气管征（图 5-2-1）。

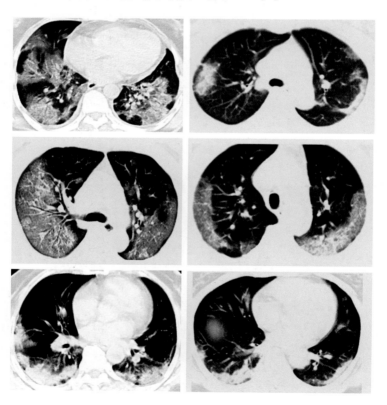

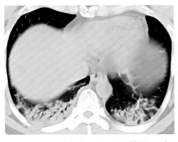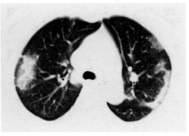

图 5-2-1　双肺叶见多发斑片状、扇形磨玻璃密度影或实变影，病灶主要分布于胸膜下，磨玻璃病灶中可见小叶间隔增厚，呈"碎石路征"，并可见增粗血管影及空气支气管征

第三节　新型冠状病毒肺炎早期不典型者 CT 表现特点

无论轻症或重症患者，病灶单发均少见，少数呈类圆形或结节状，且可见晕征或反晕征；病灶分布不以胸膜下为主，可随机分布或按血管支气管束分布；少数病例可合并胸腔积液。因此，较难与肺腺癌或其他类型病毒性肺炎相鉴别。

一、病灶形态

病灶呈类圆形、结节状改变，部分结节可见晕征（图 5-3-1）。

二、病灶性质

病灶以实变为主，少数实变病灶中可见小空洞（图 5-3-2）。

三、病灶分布

病灶单发少见，呈随机分布或按血管支气管束分布（图 5-3-3）。

四、并发症

病灶仅少数可合并胸腔积液（图 5-3-4）。

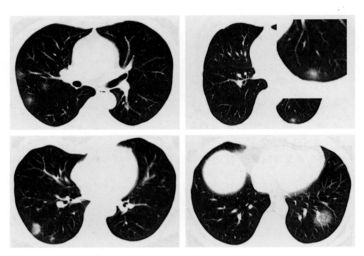

图 5-3-1　双肺叶见大小不等结节状磨玻璃高密度影，部分病灶周围可见晕征，部分病灶边界清晰

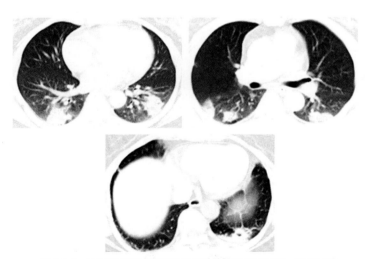

图 5-3-2　双肺叶胸膜下叶见斑片状、团片状高密度影，边界不清，部分病灶内可见小空洞影

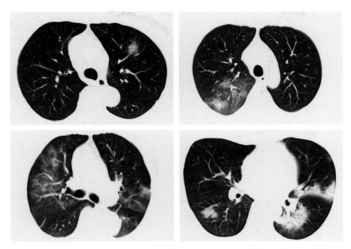

图 5-3-3　双肺叶见单发或多发斑片状磨玻璃高密度影，部分病灶沿血管支气管束分布，部分病灶呈扇形分布，边界模糊

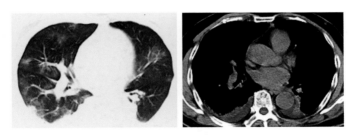

图 5-3-4　双肺叶见多发斑片状磨玻璃密度影，边界模糊；两侧胸腔见少量积液，伴有双肺下叶部分肺组织轻度膨胀不全

6

第六章

新型冠状病毒肺炎进展期肺部 CT 表现特点

新型冠状病毒肺炎进展期，一般在最初症状出现后的 5 ~ 8 天，在这一阶段，感染迅速加重，并扩展到双侧肺叶，呈弥漫性磨玻璃密度影，部分病灶实变，磨玻璃密度影与实变影或条索影共存，可伴有小叶间隔增厚等。

第一节　新型冠状病毒肺炎进展期轻症 CT 表现特点

常双侧肺叶受累，胸膜下呈非对称性分布。实变与磨玻璃病变并存，实变病变较早期增多。实变内可见空气支气管征，可见晕征或反晕征（图 6-1-1 ~ 图 6-1-4）。

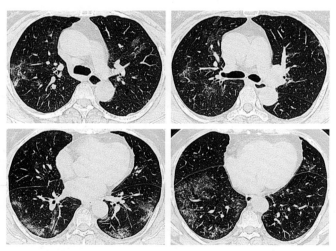

图 6-1-1　患者女性，61 岁，发热、咳嗽、胸闷 5 天，进展期轻症肺部 CT 显示双肺多发磨玻璃密度影（部分为亚实性）

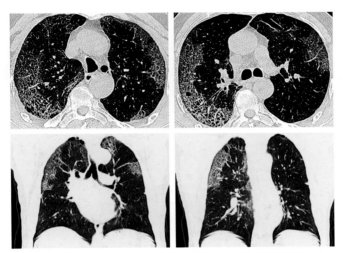

图 6-1-2　患者男性，70 岁，咳嗽、发热 1 天、进展期轻症肺部 CT
显示双肺胸膜下磨玻璃影，局部间质性病变

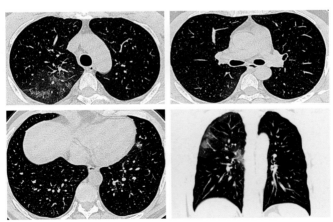

图 6-1-3　患者男性，43 岁，发热半天，进展期轻症肺部 CT 显示右
肺上叶、下叶及左肺上叶舌段磨玻璃斑片影（多肺叶受累）

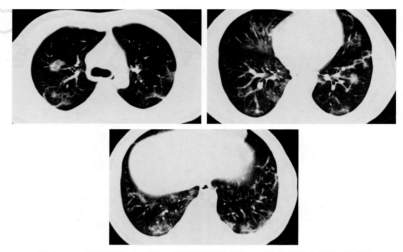

图 6-1-4　患者男性，39 岁，进展期轻症肺部 CT 显示双肺多发磨玻璃斑片影，右肺病灶可见反晕征

第二节　新型冠状病毒肺炎进展期重症 CT 表现特点

病灶分布区域增多，胸膜下分布为主，可累及多个肺叶，可由肺外围向中央进展。部分病变范围融合扩大，密度增高，呈不规则、楔形或扇形；部分病灶可多灶融合呈大片，呈双侧非对称性。支气管血管束增粗或胸膜下多灶性肺实变软组织密度影，病灶进展及变化迅速，可见亚段性肺不张，合并肺纤维化；少数可出现胸腔积液（图 6-2-1 ～ 图 6-2-12）。

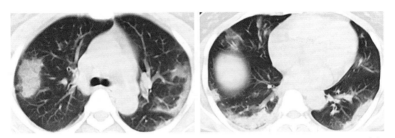

图 6-2-1　患者女性，52 岁，咳嗽、发热 10 天，进展期重症肺部 CT 显示双肺多
　　　　　发磨玻璃密度影、空气支气管征

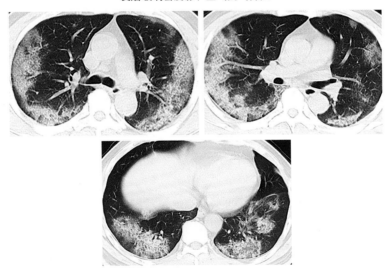

图 6-2-2　患者男性，55 岁，咳嗽伴发热 8 天，进展期重症肺部 CT 显示双肺磨
　　　　　玻璃密度影或实变影、空气支气管征，病变累及多个肺叶

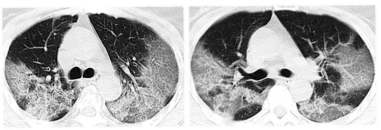

图 6-2-3　患者女性，65 岁，发热、咳嗽 11 天，进展期重症肺部 CT 显示两侧胸
　　　　　膜下大范围磨玻璃密度影，部分病灶内可见增粗血管影

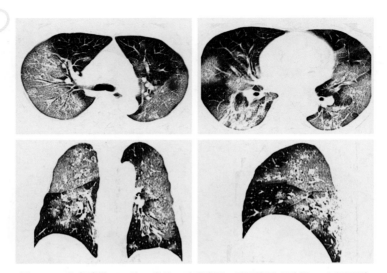

图 6-2-4　患者男性，56 岁，发热、咳嗽半天，进展期重症肺部 CT 显示双肺磨玻璃密度影、实变影或条索影，多累及肺叶，可见空气支气管征，病灶内血管增粗，双肺下叶病灶内可见肺纤维化

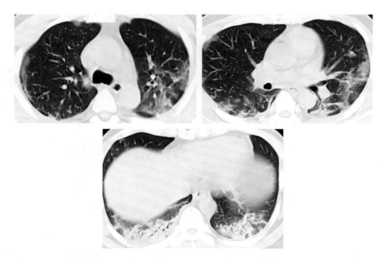

图 6-2-5　患者男性，37 岁，发热 1 天、进展期重症肺部 CT 显示双肺多发斑片，胸膜下多灶性肺实变影

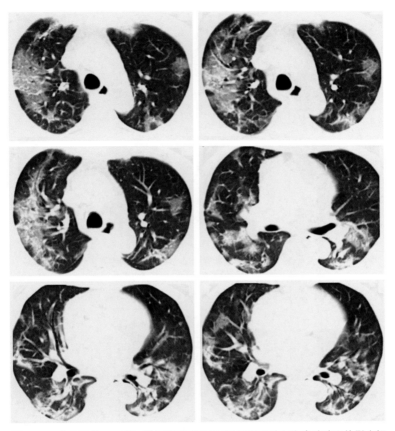

图 6-2-6　患者男性，54 岁，进展期重症肺部 CT 显示双肺多发磨玻璃斑片影（部分亚实性）、可见空气支气管征，双肺下叶病灶内可见结节和条索影

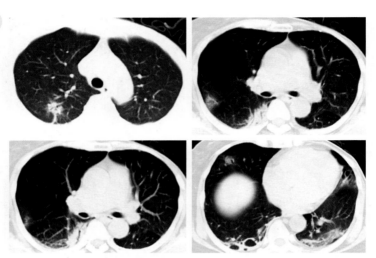

图 6-2-7　患者女性，62 岁，进展期重症肺部 CT 显示胸膜下多灶性肺实变影，
局部病灶合并纤维化

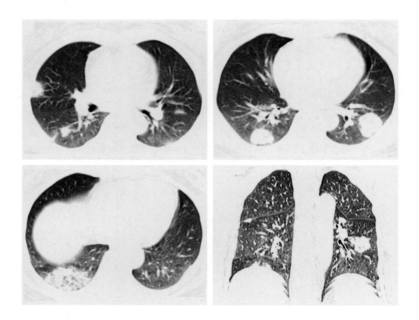

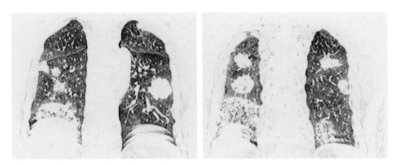

图 6-2-8 患者女性，45 岁，进展期重症肺部 CT 显示病灶分布区域增多，部分
病变融合扩大，密度增高，呈"团块样"改变

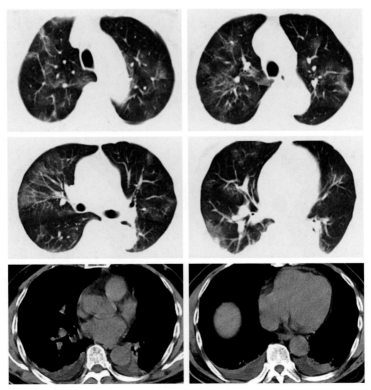

图 6-2-9 患者男性，75 岁，进展期重症肺部 CT 显示病变累及范围广，合
并少量胸腔积液

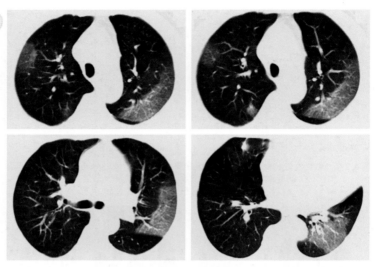

图 6-2-10　患者男性，74 岁，进展期重症肺部 CT 显示病灶分布区域增多，胸膜下分布为主，血管支气管束增粗

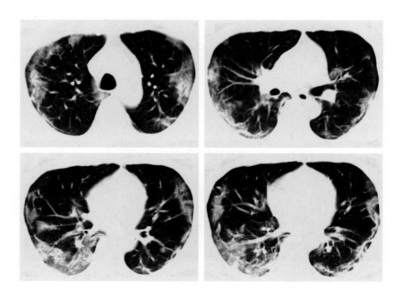

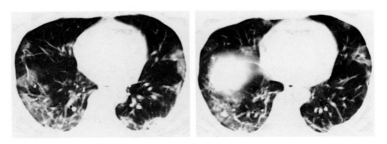

图 6-2-11　患者女性，47 岁，进展期重症肺部 CT 显示胸膜下多灶性斑片、结节影，合并纤维化，血管支气管束增粗，局部间质性改变

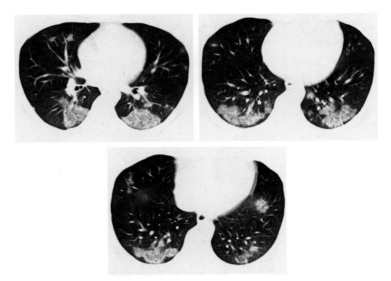

图 6-2-12　患者男性，34 岁，进展期重症肺部 CT 显示胸膜下多灶性磨玻璃影伴实变，病灶内血管增粗

第三节 新型冠状病毒肺炎进展期 不典型者 CT 表现特点

病灶呈散在斑片、条索影或片状实变影，与其他类型肺炎较难鉴别（图 6-3-1，图 6-3-2）。

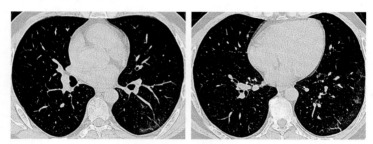

图 6-3-1 患者男性，41 岁，发热、咳嗽 3 天，进展期不典型肺部 CT 显示左肺下叶斑片、条索影

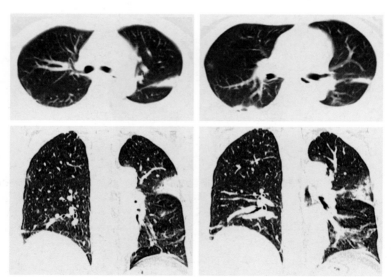

图 6-3-2 患者女性，35 岁，进展期不典型肺部 CT 显示左肺下叶片状实变影

7

第七章

新型冠状病毒肺炎高峰期
肺部 CT 表现特点

新型冠状病毒肺炎高峰期（初始症状出现后 9 ~ 13 天）的肺部 CT 表现较进展期稳定，肺内病灶的大小、数目、密度及分布范围均达到峰值，原有的磨玻璃密度增加，普遍进展为混杂密度或实变灶。此期的 CT 可表现为混杂磨玻璃密度影、"碎石路征"、实变等，实变和空气支气管征常见，伴或不伴纤维化改变等。病理学提示弥漫性肺泡损伤伴细胞纤维黏液性渗出。

轻症患者和重症患者高峰期 CT 表现在程度上有所不同。

第一节　新型冠状病毒肺炎高峰期轻症 CT 表现特点

轻症患者病变局限，可为双肺或者单肺受累，好发于胸膜下，病灶以大小不等的磨玻璃密度影或混杂密度影多见，可伴有小范围实变、纤维化趋势，长轴多与胸膜平行（图 7-1-1 ~ 图 7-1-7）。

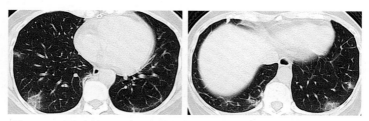

图 7-1-1　患者女性，45 岁，发热、咳嗽 2 天，有确诊患者接触史，发病第 6 天肺部 CT 显示双肺胸膜下多发磨玻璃密度影，以下叶多见，伴血管增粗，小叶间隔增厚

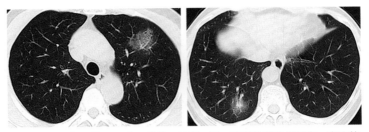

图 7-1-2　患者男性，69 岁，发热、咳嗽 1 天，有确诊患者接触史，发病第 7 天肺部 CT 显示右肺下叶及左肺上叶磨玻璃密度影，伴血管增粗、小叶间隔增厚

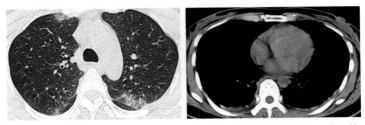

图 7-1-3　患者女性，45 岁，发热、咳嗽 4 天，有确诊患者接触史，发病第 8 天肺部 CT 显示双肺斜裂旁多发磨玻璃密度影，两侧胸前少量积液

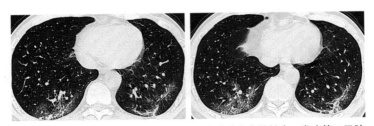

图 7-1-4　患者男性，43 岁，发热 1 天，有确诊患者接触史，发病第 7 天肺部 CT 显示双肺下叶胸膜下多发斑片状、磨玻璃密度影伴纤维化趋势，可见部分支气管扩张、小叶间隔增厚

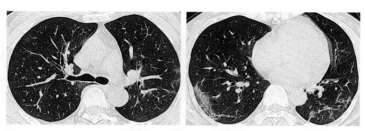

图 7-1-5　患者女性，48 岁，发热 1 天，有确诊患者接触史，发病第 12 天肺部 CT 显示双肺胸膜下多发磨玻璃密度影伴纤维化趋势，部分支气管扩张、小叶间隔增厚

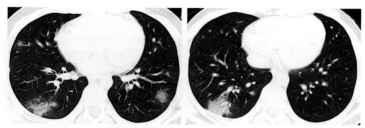

图 7-1-6　患者男性，12 岁，无症状，有确诊患者接触史，发病第 2 天肺部 CT 显示双肺胸膜下多发磨玻璃密度影，沿支气管血管束分布，可见空支气管征

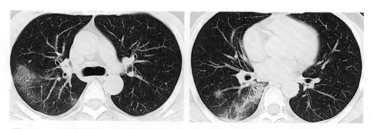

图 7-1-7　患者男性，43 岁，发热、咳嗽 1 天，有确诊患者接触史，发病第 8 天肺部 CT 显示右肺多发磨玻璃密度影伴部分实变

第二节　新型冠状病毒肺炎高峰期重症 CT 表现特点

双肺弥漫性病变多见，病情进展迅速，48 小时病灶范围增加，可达 50%。当 1/2 以上肺野被病变占据时，则出现"白肺"。病变以实变

为主，合并磨玻璃密度影，可伴多发条索状阴影。多合并其他疾病，病
情较危重（图 7-2-1 ~ 图 7-2-10）。

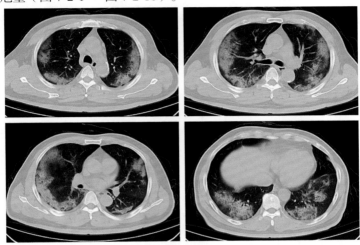

图 7-2-1　患者男性，56 岁，有确诊患者接触史，主要症状为发热、干咳，
发病第 10 天肺部 CT 显示磨玻璃密度影、"碎石路征"，广泛分布于各个肺叶，
以胸膜下为著

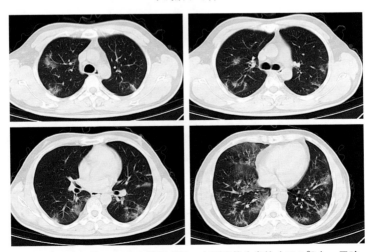

图 7-2-2　患者男性，39 岁，长居武汉，主要症状为发热（38.5 ℃）、干咳，
发病第 17 天肺部 CT 显示磨玻璃密度影、片状影或条索影，以双肺下叶为著，
胸膜下及肺内随机分布

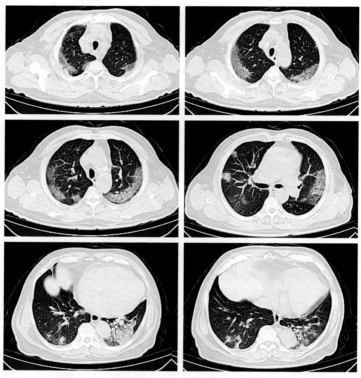

图 7-2-3　患者男性，54 岁，有确诊患者接触史，发病第 12 天肺部 CT 显示
磨玻璃密度影、小叶间隔增厚或条索影，病变范围累及胸膜下及肺内

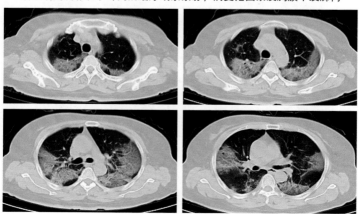

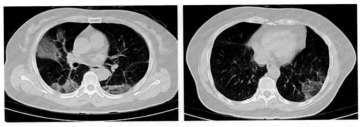

图 7-2-4　患者女性，45 岁，长居武汉，以发热、干咳为主要症状，发病第 15 天肺部 CT 显示磨玻璃密度影、"碎石路征"或条索影，双肺下叶伴实变

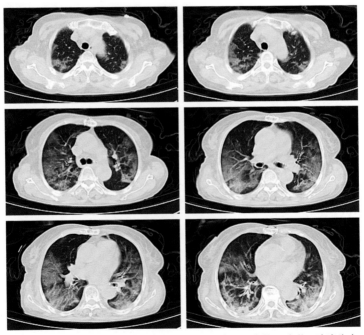

图 7-2-5　患者男性，70 岁，有确诊患者接触史，以发热、咳嗽、咳痰为主要症状，合并慢性支气管炎、肺气肿，发病第 7 天肺部 CT 显示"碎石路征"、条索影，病变以胸膜下为著

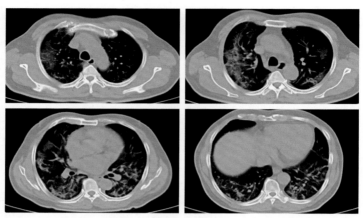

图 7-2-6　患者男性，30 岁，长居武汉，以发热、胸闷、腹泻为主要症状，发病第 4 天肺部 CT 显示磨玻璃或纤维条索影，以双肺下叶为著

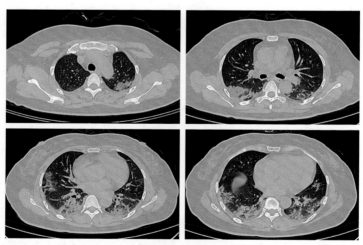

图 7-2-7　患者男性，74 岁，长居武汉，咳嗽、咳痰，无发热，发病第 18 天肺部 CT 显示磨玻璃密度影、"碎石路征"，左肺下叶伴实变

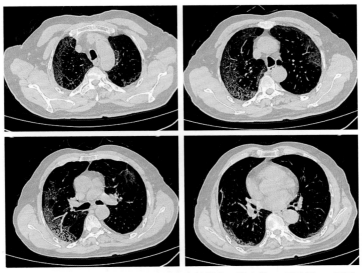

图 7-2-8　患者女性，65 岁，有确诊患者接触史，发病第 10 天肺部 CT 显示磨玻璃密度影、"碎石路征"及纤维条索影，病变累及胸膜下及肺内，以双肺上叶为主

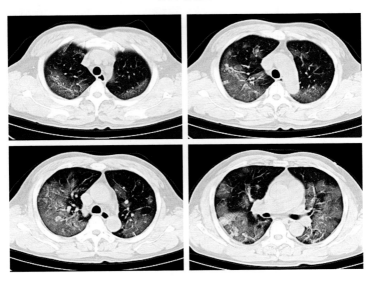

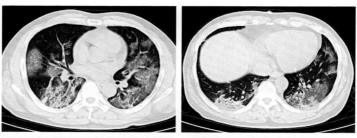

图 7-2-9　患者女性，68 岁，发热伴腹泻，发病第 16 天肺部 CT 显示磨玻璃密度影、斑片影及"碎石路征"，双肺下叶部分实变，胸膜下及肺内均出现

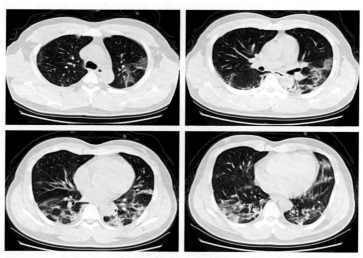

图 7-2-10　患者男性，56 岁，有确诊患者接触史，主要症状为发热、干咳，发病第 7 天肺部 CT 显示双肺弥漫分布的磨玻璃密度影及纤维条索影，部分实变

第三节　新型冠状病毒肺炎高峰期
不典型者 CT 表现特点

　　部分新型冠状病毒肺炎患者高峰期胸部 CT 表现不典型，主要有以下几种情况。

一、病灶分布

病灶分布于个别肺叶（段），呈单发混杂密度影或实变影，伴有空气支气管征、小血管网增粗及小叶间隔增厚（图 7-3-1 ~ 图 7-3-4）。

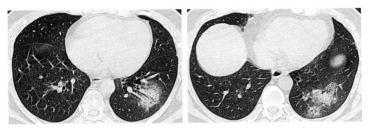

图 7-3-1　患者男性，38 岁，有确诊患者接触史，主要症状为发热、干咳，发病第 6 天肺部 CT 显示左肺下叶单发片团状实变影，伴空气支气管征、小叶间隔增厚

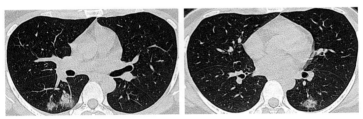

图 7-3-2　患者女性，33 岁，发热 1 天，有确诊患者接触史，发病第 11 天肺部 CT 显示双肺下叶胸膜下多发混杂磨玻璃密度影，部分病灶可见毛刺和分叶

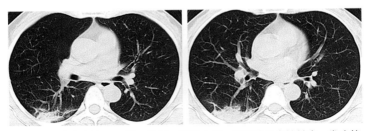

图 7-3-3　患者女性，55 岁，发热、咳嗽 1 天，有确诊患者接触史，发病第 9 天肺部 CT 显示右肺下叶胸膜下单发片团状实变影

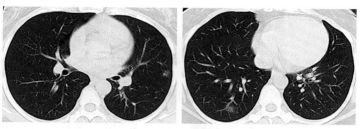

图 7-3-4　患者女性，34 岁，无症状，有确诊患者接触史，发病第 5 天肺部 CT 显示双肺胸膜下少许磨玻璃密度影

二、病灶累及

病灶累及中内带（图 7-3-5，图 7-3-6）。

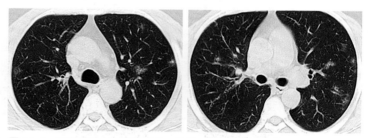

图 7-3-5　患者男性，48 岁，发热、咳嗽 3 天就诊，发病第 18 天肺部 CT 显示双肺多发磨玻璃密度影，沿支气管血管束分布，以胸膜下多见，双肺中内带亦有累及

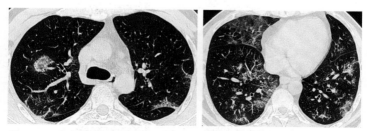

图 7-3-6　患者男性，39 岁，发热、咳嗽 1 天，发病第 14 天肺部 CT 显示双肺多发磨玻璃密度影，外中内带同时受累

8

第八章

新型冠状病毒肺炎消散期肺部 CT 表现特点

　　多见于肺炎发病后 10 天左右，部分轻症患者可提前 1 周左右。临床上感染控制，肺部病变逐渐吸收，病变范围逐渐缩小，肺实变逐渐消失演变成磨玻璃密度影，最后逐渐消失或残存部分呈条索影（图 8-1-1 ～图 8-1-4）。

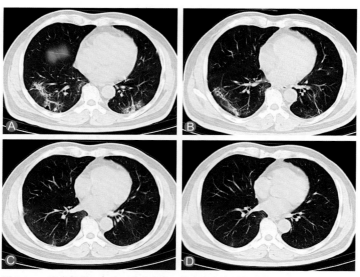

图 8-1-1　患者男性，56 岁，重症患者，有确诊患者接触史，发病第 21 天（A）、第 30 天（B）、第 46 天（C）、第 65 天（D）肺部 CT 显示双肺下叶条片状影逐渐吸收，至发病第 65 天左肺下叶病变基本消失，右肺下叶见少许磨玻璃稍高密度影

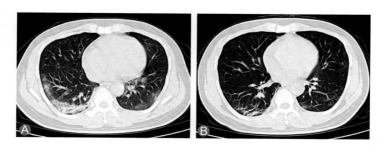

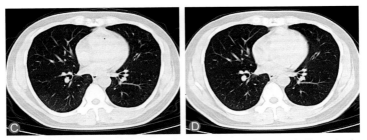

图 8-1-2　患者男性，41 岁，重症患者，长居武汉，发病第 6 天（A）、第 9 天（B）、第 15 天（C）、第 30 天（D）肺部 CT 显示双肺下叶实变影逐渐吸收，演变为条片状影，至发病第 30 天基本消失

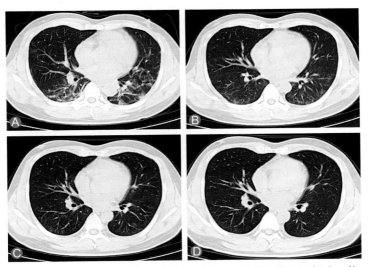

图 8-1-3　患者男性，37 岁，重症患者，长居武汉，发病第 7 天（A）、第 16 天（B）、第 22 天（C）、第 36 天（D）肺部 CT 显示双肺多发条片状影逐渐吸收，转变为磨玻璃密度影，至发病第 36 天双肺病变基本消失

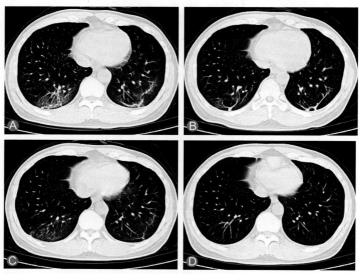

图 8-1-4　患者男性，43 岁，轻症患者，长居武汉，发病第 7 天（A）、第 10 天（B）、第 17 天（C）、第 46 天（D）肺部 CT，第 7 天表现为双肺下叶条片状影、磨玻璃密度影及"碎石路征"，第 10 天"碎石路征"基本消失，第 17 天条片状影演变为磨玻璃密度影，第 46 天双肺病变基本消失

附录一

新型冠状病毒肺炎
出院患者康复方案（试行）

为改善新型冠状病毒肺炎患者呼吸功能、躯体功能及心理功能障碍，规范康复的操作技术及流程，特制订本方案。

一、目标

改善新型冠状病毒肺炎出院患者呼吸困难症状和功能障碍，减少并发症，缓解焦虑、抑郁情绪，降低致残率，最大程度恢复日常活动能力、提高生活质量。

二、适用人群及场所

1. 人群：新型冠状病毒肺炎出院患者。

2. 场所：指定的出院后患者康复医疗机构、隔离场所、养老院、社区、家庭。

三、主要内容

（一）需开展康复治疗的功能障碍

1. 呼吸功能障碍：表现为咳嗽、咳痰、呼吸困难、活动后气短，可伴有呼吸肌无力及肺功能受损等。

2. 躯体功能障碍：表现为全身乏力、易疲劳、肌肉酸痛，部分可伴有肌肉萎缩、肌力下降等。

3. 心理功能障碍：有恐惧、愤怒、焦虑、抑郁等情绪问题。

4. 日常生活活动能力及社会参与能力障碍：无法独立完成穿脱衣、如厕、洗澡等。无法实现正常的人际交往和无法重返工作岗位。

（二）康复功能评估

1. 呼吸功能评估：采用呼吸困难指数量表（mMRC）等进行评估，有条件的地区或机构建议行肺功能检查。

2. 躯体功能评估：采用 Borg 自觉疲劳量表、徒手肌力检查等进行评估。

3.心理功能评估：采用抑郁自评量表（SDS）、焦虑自评量表（SAS）、匹兹堡睡眠问卷等进行评估。

4.日常生活活动能力评估：采用改良巴氏指数评定表等进行评估。

5.六分钟步行试验：要求患者在平直走廊里尽可能快地行走，测定六分钟的步行距离，最小折返距离≥ 30 m。

四、康复治疗方法

（一）呼吸功能训练

主动循环呼吸技术（active cycle of breathing techniques，ACBT）：一个循环周期由呼吸控制、胸廓扩张运动和用力呼气技术 3 个部分组成。呼吸控制阶段指导患者用放松的方法以正常的潮气量进行呼吸，鼓励肩部及上胸部保持放松，下胸部及腹部主动收缩，以膈肌呼吸模式完成呼吸，该阶段持续时间应与患者对放松的需求相适应。胸廓扩张阶段强调吸气，指导患者深吸气到吸气储备量，屏息 1 ~ 2 秒，然后被动而轻松地呼气。用力呼气阶段为穿插呼吸控制及呵气。呵气是一种快速但不用最大努力的呼气，过程中声门应保持开放。利用呵气技巧进行排痰，代替咳嗽降低呼吸肌做功。注意在呵气过程中用口罩遮挡。

呼吸模式训练：包括调整呼吸节奏（吸∶呼 =1∶2）、腹式呼吸训练、缩唇呼吸训练等。

呼吸康复操：根据患者体力情况进行卧位、坐位及站立位的颈屈伸、扩胸、转身、旋腰、侧躯、蹲起、抬腿、开腿、踝泵等系列运动。

（二）躯体功能训练

有氧运动：针对患者合并的基础疾病和遗留功能障碍问题制定有氧运动处方，包括踏步、慢走、快走、慢跑、游泳、太极拳、八段锦等运动形式。以运动后第 2 天不出现疲劳的运动强度为宜，从低强度开始，循序渐进，每次 20 ~ 30 分钟，每周 3 ~ 5 次。对于容易疲劳的患者可采取间歇运动形式进行。餐后 1 小时后开始。

力量训练：使用沙袋、哑铃、弹力带或瓶装水等进行渐进抗阻训练，每组 15 ~ 20 个动作，每天 1 ~ 2 组，每周 3 ~ 5 天。

（三）心理康复干预

设计可产生愉悦效应及转移注意力的作业疗法，达成调整情绪、疏解压力的目的。通过专业心理学培训的护理人员和康复治疗师也可以开展专业的心理咨询，包括正念放松治疗和认知行为治疗。注意慎用让患者重复叙述创伤经历的方法，以免造成重复伤害。如出现精神障碍，建议精神专科介入。

（四）日常生活活动能力训练

对患者进行日常生活活动指导。主要是节能技术指导，将穿脱衣、如厕、洗澡等日常生活活动动作分解成小节间歇进行，随着体力恢复再连贯完成，逐步恢复至正常。

五、有关注意事项

（一）禁忌证

如患者出现以下情况之一，不建议开展上述康复治疗。

1. 静态心率＞ 100 次 / 分。

2. 血压＜ 90/60 mmHg、血压＞ 140/90 mmHg 或血压波动超过基线 20 mmHg，并伴有明显头晕、头痛等不适症状。

3. 血氧饱和度≤ 95%。

4. 合并其他不适合运动的疾病。

（二）停止治疗

当患者在治疗过程中出现以下情况，应立即停止上述康复治疗，重新评估并调整治疗方案。

1. 出现明显疲劳，休息后不能缓解。

2. 出现胸闷、胸痛、呼吸困难、剧烈咳嗽、头晕、头痛、视物不清、心悸、大汗、站立不稳等。

3. 当患者合并有肺动脉高压、充血性心力衰竭、深静脉血栓、不稳定的骨折等疾病则应与专科医师咨询相关注意事项后再开始呼吸康复治疗。

4. 高龄患者常伴有多种基础疾病，体质较差，对康复训练的耐受能力较差，康复治疗前应进行综合评估，康复训练应从小剂量开始，循序渐进，避免出现训练损伤及其他严重并发症。

5. 重型、危重型患者出院后，视当地康复医疗工作实际情况，可在指定的康复医疗机构、基层医疗卫生机构进行出院后康复。轻型、普通型患者出院后，社区及居家应适当休息、适当运动，尽最大可能恢复体能、体质和免疫能力。

新型冠状病毒肺炎
诊疗方案（试行第七版）

2019 年 12 月以来，湖北省武汉市出现了新型冠状病毒肺炎疫情，随着疫情的蔓延，我国其他地区及境外多个国家也相继发现了此类病例。该病作为急性呼吸道传染病已纳入《中华人民共和国传染病防治法》规定的乙类传染病，按甲类传染病管理。通过采取一系列预防控制和医疗救治措施，我国境内疫情上升的势头得到一定程度的遏制，大多数省份疫情缓解，但境外的发病人数呈上升态势。随着对疾病临床表现、病理认识的深入和诊疗经验的积累，为进一步加强对该病的早诊早治，提高治愈率，降低病亡率，最大可能避免医院感染，同时提醒注意境外输入性病例导致的传播和扩散，并对《新型冠状病毒肺炎诊疗方案（试行第六版）》进行修订，形成了《新型冠状病毒肺炎诊疗方案（试行第七版）》。

一、病原学特点

新型冠状病毒属于 β 属的冠状病毒，有包膜，颗粒呈圆形或椭圆形，常为多形性，直径 60 ~ 140 nm。其基因特征与 SARS-CoV 和 MERS-CoV 有明显区别。目前研究显示与蝙蝠 SARS 样冠状病毒（bat-SL-CoVZC45）同源性达 85% 以上。体外分离培养时，新型冠状病毒在 96 个小时左右即可在人呼吸道上皮细胞内发现，而在 Vero E6 和 Huh-7 细胞系中分离培养约需 6 天。

对冠状病毒理化特性的认识多来自对 SARS-CoV 和 MERS-CoV 的研究。病毒对紫外线和热敏感，56℃ 30 分钟、乙醚、75% 乙醇、含氯消毒剂、过氧乙酸和氯仿等脂溶剂均可有效灭活病毒，氯己定不能有效灭活病毒。

二、流行病学特点

（一）传染源

目前所见传染源主要是新型冠状病毒感染的患者。无症状感染者也可能成为传染源。

（二）传播途径

经呼吸道飞沫和密切接触传播是主要的传播途径。在相对封闭的环境中长时间暴露于高浓度气溶胶情况下存在经气溶胶传播的可能。由于在粪便及尿中可分离到新型冠状病毒，应注意粪便及尿对环境污染造成气溶胶或接触传播。

（三）易感人群

人群普遍易感。

三、病理改变

根据目前有限的尸检和穿刺组织病理观察结果总结如下。

（一）肺

肺呈不同程度的实变。

肺泡腔内见浆液、纤维蛋白性渗出物及透明膜形成；渗出细胞主要为单核和巨噬细胞，易见多核巨细胞。Ⅱ型肺泡上皮细胞显著增生，部分细胞脱落。Ⅱ型肺泡上皮细胞和巨噬细胞内可见包涵体。肺泡隔血管充血、水肿，可见单核和淋巴细胞浸润及血管内透明血栓形成。肺组织灶性出血、坏死，可出现出血性梗死。部分肺泡腔渗出物机化和肺间质纤维化。

肺内支气管黏膜部分上皮脱落，腔内可见黏液及黏液栓形成。少数肺泡过度充气、肺泡隔断裂或囊腔形成。

电镜下支气管黏膜上皮和Ⅱ型肺泡上皮细胞胞质内可见冠状病毒颗粒。免疫组化染色显示部分肺泡上皮和巨噬细胞呈新型冠状病毒抗原阳性，RT-PCR检测新型冠状病毒核酸阳性。

（二）脾、肺门淋巴结和骨髓

脾明显缩小。淋巴细胞数量明显减少，灶性出血和坏死，脾内巨噬细胞增生并可见吞噬现象；淋巴结淋巴细胞数量较少，可见坏死。免疫组化染色显示脾和淋巴结内 CD4$^+$T 和 CD8$^+$T 细胞均减少。骨髓三系细胞数量减少。

（三）心血管

心肌细胞可见变性、坏死，间质内可见少数单核细胞、淋巴细胞和 / 或中性粒细胞浸润。部分血管内皮脱落、内膜炎症及血栓形成。

（四）肝和胆囊

体积增大，暗红色。肝细胞变性、灶性坏死伴中性粒细胞浸润；肝血窦充血，汇管区见淋巴细胞和单核细胞细胞浸润，微血栓形成。胆囊高度充盈。

（五）肾

肾小球球囊腔内见蛋白性渗出物，肾小管上皮变性、脱落，可见透明管型。间质充血，可见微血栓和灶性纤维化。

（六）其他器官

脑组织充血、水肿，部分神经元变性。肾上腺见灶性坏死。食管、胃和肠管黏膜上皮不同程度变性、坏死、脱落。

四、临床特点

（一）临床表现

基于目前的流行病学调查，潜伏期 1 ~ 4 天，多为 3 ~ 7 天。

以发热、干咳、乏力为主要表现。少数患者伴有鼻塞、流涕、咽痛、肌痛和腹泻等症状。重症患者多在发病一周后出现呼吸困难和 / 或低氧血症，严重者可快速进展为急性呼吸窘迫综合征、脓毒症休克、难以纠正的代谢性酸中毒和出凝血功能障碍及多器官功能衰竭等。值得注意的是重型、危重型患者病程中可为中低热，甚至无明显发热。

部分儿童及新生儿病例症状可不典型，表现为呕吐、腹泻等消化道症状或仅表现为精神弱、呼吸急促。

轻型患者仅表现为低热、轻微乏力等，无肺炎表现。

从目前收治的病例情况看，多数患者预后良好，少数患者病情危重。老年人和有慢性基础疾病者预后较差。患有新型冠状病毒肺炎的孕产妇临床过程与同龄患者相近。儿童病例症状相对较轻。

（二）实验室检查

1. 一般检查

发病早期外周血白细胞总数正常或减少，可见淋巴细胞计数减少，部分患者可出现肝酶、乳酸脱氢酶（LDH）、肌酶和肌红蛋白增高；部分危重者可见肌钙蛋白增高。多数患者 CRP 和 ESR 升高，降钙素原正常。严重者 D- 二聚体升高、外周血淋巴细胞进行性减少。重型、危重型患者常有炎症因子升高。

2. 病原学及血清学检查

（1）病原学检查：采用 RT-PCR 和 / 或 NGS 方法在鼻咽拭子、痰和其他下呼吸道分泌物、血液、粪便等标本中可检测出新型冠状病毒核酸。检测下呼吸道标本（痰或气道抽取物）更加准确。标本采集后尽快送检。

（2）血清学检查：新型冠状病毒特异性 IgM 抗体多在发病 3 ～ 5 天后开始出现阳性，IgG 抗体滴度恢复期较急性期有 4 倍及以上增高。

（三）胸部影像学

早期呈现多发小斑片影及间质改变，以肺外带明显。进而发展为双肺多发磨玻璃影、浸润影，严重者可出现肺实变，胸腔积液少见。

五、诊断标准

（一）疑似病例

结合下述流行病学史和临床表现综合分析。

1. 流行病学史

（1）发病前 14 天内有武汉市及周边地区，或其他有病例报告社区的旅行史或居住史。

（2）发病前 14 天内与新型冠状病毒感染者（核酸检测阳性者）有接触史。

（3）发病前 14 天内曾接触过来自武汉市及周边地区，或来自有病例报告社区的发热或有呼吸道症状的患者。

（4）聚集性发病（2 周内在小范围如家庭、办公室、学校班级等场所，出现 2 例及以上发热和 / 或呼吸道症状的病例）。

2. 临床表现

（1）发热和 / 或呼吸道症状。

（2）具有上述新型冠状病毒肺炎影像学特征。

（3）发病早期白细胞总数正常或降低，淋巴细胞计数正常或减少。

有流行病学史中的任何一条，且符合临床表现中任意 2 条。无明确流行病学史的，符合临床表现中的 3 条，可判定为疑似病例。

（二）确诊病例

疑似病例同时具备以下病原学或血清学证据之一者。

（1）实时荧光 RT-PCR 检测新型冠状病毒核酸阳性。

（2）病毒基因测序，与已知的新型冠状病毒高度同源。

（3）血清新型冠状病毒特异性 IgM 抗体和 IgG 抗体阳性；血清新型冠状病毒特异性 IgG 抗体由阴性转为阳性或恢复期较急性期 4 倍及以上升高。

六、临床分型

（一）轻型

临床症状轻微，影像学未见肺炎表现。

（二）普通型

具有发热、呼吸道等症状，影像学可见肺炎表现。

（三）重型

1. 成年人符合下列任何一条者。

（1）出现气促，RR ≥ 30 次 / 分。

（2）静息状态下，指氧饱和度 ≤ 93%。

（3）动脉血氧分压（PaO_2）/ 吸氧浓度（FiO_2） ≤ 300 mmHg（1 mmHg=0.133 kPa）。

高海拔（海拔超过 1000 m）地区应根据以下公式对 PaO_2/FiO_2 进行校正：$PaO_2/FiO_2 ×$ [大气压（mmHg）/760]。

肺部影像学显示 24 ~ 48 小时内病灶明显进展 > 50% 者按重型管理。

2. 儿童符合下列任何一条者。

（1）出现气促（< 2 个月龄，RR ≥ 60 次 / 分；2 ~ 12 个月龄，RR ≥ 50 次 / 分；1 ~ 5 岁，RR ≥ 40 次 / 分；> 5 岁，RR ≥ 30 次 / 分），除外发热和哭闹的影响。

（2）静息状态下氧饱和度 ≤ 92%。

（3）辅助呼吸（呻吟、鼻翼扇动、三凹征），发绀，间歇性呼吸暂停。

（4）出现嗜睡、惊厥。

（5）拒食或喂养困难，有脱水现象。

（四）危重型

符合以下情况之一者。

1.出现呼吸衰竭，且需要机械通气。

2.出现休克。

3.合并其他器官功能衰竭需 ICU 监护治疗。

七、重型、危重型临床预警指标

（一）成年人

1.外周血淋巴细胞进行性下降。

2.外周血炎症因子如 IL-6、CRP 进行性上升。

3.乳酸进行性升高。

4.肺内病变在短期内迅速进展。

（二）儿童

1.呼吸频率增快。

2.精神反应差、嗜睡。

3.乳酸进行性升高。

4.影像学显示双侧或多肺叶浸润、胸腔积液或短期内病变快速进展。

5.3 个月龄以下的婴儿或有基础疾病（先天性心脏病、支气管肺发育不良、呼吸道畸形、异常血红蛋白、重度营养不良等），有免疫缺陷或低下（长期使用免疫抑制剂）。

八、鉴别诊断

1. 新型冠状病毒感染轻型表现需与其他病毒引起的上呼吸道感染相鉴别。

2. 新型冠状病毒肺炎主要与流感病毒、腺病毒、呼吸道合胞病毒等其他已知病毒性肺炎及肺炎支原体感染鉴别，尤其是对疑似病例要尽可能采取包括快速抗原检测和多重 PCR 核酸检测等方法，对常见呼吸道病原体进行检测。

3. 还要与非感染性疾病，如血管炎、皮肌炎和机化性肺炎等鉴别。

九、病例的发现与报告

各级各类医疗机构的医务人员发现符合病例定义的疑似病例后，应当立即进行单人间隔离治疗，院内专家会诊或主诊医师会诊，仍考虑疑似病例者，在 2 小时内进行网络直报，并采集标本进行新型冠状病毒核酸检测，同时在确保转运安全前提下立即将疑似病例转运至定点医院。与新型冠状病毒感染者有密切接触的患者，即便常见呼吸道病原检测阳性，也建议及时进行新型冠状病毒病原学检测。

疑似病例连续两次新型冠状病毒核酸检测阴性（采样时间至少间隔 24 小时）且发病 7 天后新型冠状病毒特异性抗体 IgM 和 IgG 仍为阴性可排除疑似病例诊断。

十、治疗

（一）根据病情确定治疗场所

1. 疑似及确诊病例应在具备有效隔离条件和防护条件的定点医院隔离治疗，疑似病例应单人单间隔离治疗，确诊病例可多人收治在同一病室。

2. 危重型病例应当尽早收入 ICU 治疗。

（二）一般治疗

1. 卧床休息，加强支持治疗，保证充分热量；注意水、电解质平衡，维持内环境稳定；密切监测生命体征、指氧饱和度等。

2. 根据病情监测血常规、尿常规、CRP、生化指标（肝酶、心肌酶、肾功能等）、凝血功能、动脉血气分析、胸部影像学等。有条件者可行细胞因子检测。

3. 及时给予有效氧疗措施，包括鼻导管、面罩给氧和经鼻高流量氧疗。有条件可采用氢氧混合吸入气（H_2/O_2：66.6%/33.3%）治疗。

4. 抗病毒治疗：可试用 α - 干扰素（成年人每次 500 万单位或相当剂量，加入灭菌注射用水 2 mL，每日 2 次雾化吸入）、洛匹那韦 / 利托那韦（成年人 200 mg/50 mg，每次 2 粒，每日 2 次，疗程不超过 10 天）、利巴韦林（建议与干扰素或洛匹那韦 / 利托那韦联合应用，成年人每次 500 mg，每日 2 ~ 3 次静脉输注，疗程不超过 10 天）、磷酸氯喹（18 ~ 65 岁成年人，体重大于 50 公斤者，每次 500 mg，每日 2 次，疗程 7 天；体重小于 50 公斤者，第 1 ~ 2 天每次 500 mg，每日 2 次，第 3 ~ 7 天每次 500 mg，每日 1 次）、阿比多尔（成年人 200 mg，每日 3 次，疗程不超过 10 天）。要注意上述药物的不良反应、禁忌证（如患有心脏疾病者禁用氯喹）及与其他药物的相互作用等问题。在临床应用中进一步评价目前所试用药物的疗效。不建议同时应用 3 种及以上抗病毒药物，出现不可耐受的毒副作用时应停止使用相关药物。对孕产妇患者的治疗应考虑妊娠周数，尽可能选择对胎儿影响较小的药物，以及是否终止妊娠后再进行治疗等问题，并知情告知。

5. 抗菌药物治疗：避免盲目或不恰当使用抗菌药物，尤其是联合使用广谱抗菌药物。

（三）重型、危重型病例的治疗

1. 治疗原则

在对症治疗的基础上，积极防治并发症，治疗基础疾病，预防继发感染，及时进行器官功能支持。

2. 呼吸支持

（1）氧疗：重型患者应当接受鼻导管或面罩吸氧，并及时评估呼吸窘迫和 / 或低氧血症是否缓解。

（2）高流量鼻导管氧疗或无创机械通气：当患者接受标准氧疗后呼吸窘迫和 / 或低氧血症无法缓解时，可考虑使用高流量鼻导管氧疗或无创通气。若短时间（1 ~ 2 小时）内病情无改善甚至恶化，应当及时进行气管插管和有创机械通气。

（3）有创机械通气：建议采用肺保护性通气策略，即小潮气量（6 ~ 8 mL/kg 理想体重）和低水平气道平台压力（≤ 30 cmH$_2$O）进行机械通气，以减少呼吸机相关肺损伤。在保证气道平台压为 35 cmH$_2$O 时，可适当采用高 PEEP，保持气道温化、湿化，避免长时间镇静，早期唤醒患者并进行肺康复治疗。较多患者存在人机不同步，应当及时使用镇静及肌松剂。根据气道分泌物情况，选择密闭式吸痰，必要时行支气管镜检查采取相应治疗。

（4）挽救治疗：对于严重 ARDS 患者，建议进行肺复张。在人力资源充足的情况下，每天应当进行 12 小时以上的俯卧位通气。俯卧位机械通气效果不佳者，如条件允许，应当尽快考虑 ECMO。其相关指征：①在 FiO$_2$ > 90% 时，氧合指数 < 80 mmHg，持续 3 ~ 4 小时以上；②气道平台压 ≥ 35 cmH$_2$O 单纯呼吸衰竭患者，首选 VV-ECMO 模式；若需要循环支持，则选用 VA-ECMO 模式。在基础疾病得以控制，心肺功能有恢复迹象时，可开始撤机试验。

3. 循环支持

在充分液体复苏的基础上，改善微循环，使用血管活性药物，密切监测患者血压、心率和尿量的变化，以及动脉血气分析中乳酸和碱剩余，必要时进行无创或有创血流动力学监测，如超声多普勒法、超声心动图、有创血压或持续心排血量监测。在救治过程中，注意液体平衡策略，避免过量和不足。

如果发现患者心率突发增加大于基础值的 20% 或血压下降大于基础值 20% 以上时，若伴有皮肤灌注不良和尿量减少等表现时，应密切观察患者是否存在脓毒症休克、消化道出血或心功能衰竭等情况。

4. 肾功能衰竭和肾替代治疗

危重症患者的肾功能损伤应积极寻找导致肾功能损伤的原因，如低灌注和药物等因素。对于肾衰竭患者的治疗应注重体液平衡、酸碱平衡和电解质平衡，在营养支持治疗方面应注意氮平衡、热量和微量元素等补充。重症患者可选择连续性肾替代治疗（continuous renal replacement therapy，CRRT）。其指征包括：①高钾血症；②酸中毒；③肺水肿或水负荷过重；④多器官功能不全时的液体管理。

5. 康复者血浆治疗

适用于病情进展较快、重型和危重型患者。用法用量参考《新冠肺炎康复者恢复期血浆临床治疗方案（试行第二版）》。

6. 血液净化治疗

血液净化系统包括血浆置换、吸附、灌流、血液 / 血浆滤过等，能清除炎症因子，阻断"细胞因子风暴"，从而减轻炎症反应对机体的损伤，可用于重型、危重型患者细胞因子风暴早中期的救治。

7. 免疫治疗

对于双肺广泛病变者及重型患者，且实验室检测 IL-6 水平升高者，可试用托珠单抗治疗。首次剂量 4 ~ 8 mg/kg，推荐剂量为 400 mg、0.9% 生理盐水稀释至 100 mL，输注时间大于 1 小时；首次用药疗效不佳者，可在 12 小时后追加应用一次（剂量同前），累计给药次数最多为 2 次，单次最大剂量不超过 800 mg。注意过敏反应，有结核等活动性感染者禁用。

8. 其他治疗措施

对于氧合指标进行性恶化、影像学进展迅速、机体炎症反应过度激活状态的患者，酌情短期内（3 ~ 5 日）使用糖皮质激素，建议剂量不超过相当于甲泼尼龙 1 ~ 2 mg/（kg·d），应当注意较大剂量糖皮质激素由于其免疫抑制作用，会延缓对冠状病毒的清除；可静脉给予血必净每次 100 mL，每日 2 次；可使用肠道微生态调节剂，维持肠道微生态平衡，预防继发细菌感染。

儿童重型、危重型病例可酌情考虑给予静脉滴注丙种球蛋白。

患有重型或危重型新型冠状病毒肺炎的孕妇应积极终止妊娠，剖腹产为首选。

患者常存在焦虑恐惧情绪，应当加强心理疏导。

（四）中医治疗

本病属于中医"疫"病范畴，病因为感受"疫戾"之气，各地可根据病情、当地气候特点及不同体质等情况，参照下列方案进行辨证论治。涉及到超药典剂量，应当在医师指导下使用。

1. 医学观察期

（1）临床表现 1：乏力伴胃肠不适。

推荐中成药：藿香正气胶囊（丸、水、口服液）。

（2）临床表现 2：乏力伴发热。

推荐中成药：金花清感颗粒、连花清瘟胶囊（颗粒）、疏风解毒胶囊（颗粒）。

2. 临床治疗期（确诊病例）

（1）清肺排毒汤

适用范围：结合多地医师临床观察，适用于轻型、普通型、重型患者，在危重型患者救治中可结合患者实际情况合理使用。

基础方剂：麻黄 9 g、炙甘草 6 g、杏仁 9 g、生石膏 15～30 g（先煎）、桂枝 9 g、泽泻 9 g、猪苓 9 g、白术 9 g、茯苓 15 g、柴胡 16 g、黄芩 6 g、姜半夏 9 g、生姜 9 g、紫菀 9 g、款冬花 9 g、射干 9 g、细辛 6 g、山药 12 g、枳实 6 g、陈皮 6 g、藿香 9 g。

服法：传统中药饮片，水煎服。每日 1 剂，早晚各 1 次（饭后 40 分钟），温服，3 剂一个疗程。

如有条件，每次服完药可加服大米汤半碗，舌干津液亏虚者可多服至一碗（注：如患者不发热则生石膏的用量要小，发热或壮热可加大生石膏用量）。若症状好转而未痊愈则服用第二个疗程，若患者有特殊情况或其他基础病，第二疗程可以根据实际情况修改处方，症状消失则停药。

处方来源：国家卫生健康委办公厅国家中医药管理局办公室《关于推荐在中西医结合救治新型冠状病毒感染的肺炎中使用"清肺排毒汤"的通知》（国中医药办医政函〔2020〕22 号）。

（2）轻型

※ 寒湿郁肺证

临床表现：发热，乏力，周身酸痛，咳嗽，咯痰，胸紧憋气，纳呆，恶心，呕吐，大便黏腻不爽。舌质淡胖齿痕或淡红，苔白厚腐腻或白腻，脉濡或滑。

推荐处方：生麻黄 6 g、生石膏 15 g、杏仁 9 g、羌活 15 g、葶苈子 15 g、贯众 9 g、地龙 15 g、徐长卿 15 g、藿香 15 g、佩兰 9 g、苍术 15 g、茯苓 45 g、生白术 30 g、焦三仙各 9 g、厚朴 15 g、焦槟榔 9 g、煨草果 9 g、生姜 15 g。

服法：每日 1 剂，水煎 600 mL，分 3 次服用，早中晚各 1 次，饭前服用。

※ 湿热蕴肺证

临床表现：低热或不发热，微恶寒，乏力，头身困重，肌肉酸痛，干咳痰少，咽痛，口干不欲多饮，或伴有胸闷脘痞，无汗或汗出不畅，或见呕恶纳呆，便溏或大便黏滞不爽。舌淡红，苔白厚腻或薄黄，脉滑数或濡。

推荐处方：槟榔 10 g、草果 10 g、厚朴 10 g、知母 10 g、黄芩 10 g、柴胡 10 g、赤芍 10 g、连翘 15 g、青蒿 10 g（后下）、苍术 10 g、大青叶 10 g、生甘草 5 g。

服法：每日 1 剂，水煎 400 mL，分 2 次服用，早晚各 1 次。

（3）普通型

※ 湿毒郁肺证

临床表现：发热，咳嗽痰少，或有黄痰，憋闷气促，腹胀，便秘不畅。舌质暗红，舌体胖，苔黄腻或黄燥，脉滑数或弦滑。

推荐处方：生麻黄 6 g、苦杏仁 15 g、生石膏 30 g、生薏苡仁 30 g、苍术 10 g、藿香 15 g、青蒿 12 g、虎杖 20 g、马鞭草 30 g、干芦根 30 g、葶苈子 15 g、化橘红 15 g、生甘草 10 g。

服法：每日 1 剂，水煎 400 mL，分 2 次服用，早晚各 1 次。

※ 寒湿阻肺证

临床表现：低热，身热不扬，或未热，干咳，少痰，倦怠乏力，胸闷，脘痞，或呕恶，便溏。舌质淡或淡红，苔白或白腻，脉濡。

推荐处方：苍术 15 g、陈皮 10 g、厚朴 10 g、藿香 10 g、草果 6 g、生麻黄 6 g、羌活 10 g、生姜 10 g、槟榔 10 g。

服法：每日 1 剂，水煎 400 mL，分 2 次服用，早晚各 1 次。

（4）重型

※ 疫毒闭肺证

临床表现：发热面红，咳嗽，痰黄黏少，或痰中带血，喘憋气促，疲乏倦怠，口干苦黏，恶心不食，大便不畅，小便短赤。舌红，苔黄腻，脉滑数。

推荐处方：化湿败毒方。

基础方剂：生麻黄 6 g、杏仁 9 g、生石膏 15 g、甘草 3 g、藿香 10 g（后下）、厚朴 10 g、苍术 15 g、草果 10 g、法半夏 9 g、茯苓 15 g、生大黄 5 g（后下）、生黄芪 10 g、葶苈子 10 g、赤芍 10 g。

服法：每日 1 ～ 2 剂，水煎服，每次 100 ～ 200 mL，每日 2 ～ 4 次，口服或鼻饲。

※ 气营两燔证

临床表现：大热烦渴，喘憋气促，谵语神昏，视物错瞀，或发斑疹，或吐血、衄血，或四肢抽搐。舌绛少苔或无苔，脉沉细数，或浮大而数。

推荐处方：生石膏 30 ～ 60 g（先煎）、知母 30 g、生地黄 30 ～ 60 g、水牛角 30 g（先煎）、赤芍 30 g、玄参 30 g、连翘 15 g、丹皮 15 g、黄连 6 g、淡竹叶 12 g、葶苈子 15 g、生甘草 6 g。

服法：每日 1 剂，水煎服，先煎石膏、水牛角后下诸药，每次 100 ～ 200 mL，每日 2 ～ 4 次，口服或鼻饲。

推荐中成药：喜炎平注射液、血必净注射液、热毒宁注射液、痰热清注射液、醒脑静注射液。功效相近的药物根据个体情况可选择一种，也可根据临床症状联合使用两种。中药注射剂可与中药汤剂联合使用。

（5）危重型

※ 内闭外脱证

临床表现：呼吸困难、动辄气喘或需要机械通气，伴神昏，烦躁，汗出肢冷，舌质紫暗，苔厚腻或燥，脉浮大无根。

推荐处方：人参 15 g、黑顺片 10 g（先煎）、山茱萸 15 g，送服苏合香丸或安宫牛黄丸。

出现机械通气伴腹胀便秘或大便不畅者，可用生大黄 5 ~ 10 g；出现人机不同步时，在使用镇静和肌松剂的情况下，可用生大黄 5 ~ 10 g 和芒硝 5 ~ 10 g。

推荐中成药：血必净注射液、热毒宁注射液、痰热清注射液、醒脑静注射液、参附注射液、生脉注射液、参麦注射液。功效相近的药物根据个体情况可选择一种，也可根据临床症状联合使用两种。中药注射剂可与中药汤剂联合使用。

注：重型和危重型中药注射剂推荐用法。

中药注射剂的使用遵照药品说明书从小剂量开始、逐步辨证调整的原则，推荐用法如下。

（1）病毒感染或合并轻度细菌感染：0.9% 氯化钠注射液 250 mL 加喜炎平注射液 100 mg，每日 2 次。或 0.9% 氯化钠注射液 250 mL 加热毒宁注射液 20 mL，或 0.9% 氯化钠注射液 250 mL 加痰热清注射液 40 mL，每日 2 次。

（2）高热伴意识障碍：0.9% 氯化钠注射液 250 mL 加醒脑静注射液 20 mL，每日 2 次。

（3）全身炎症反应综合征和／或多脏器功能衰竭：0.9% 氯化钠注射液 250 mL 加血必净注射液 100 mL，每日 2 次。

（4）免疫抑制：葡萄糖注射液 250 mL 加参麦注射液 100 mL 或生脉注射液 20 ~ 60 mL，每日 2 次。

（6）恢复期

※ 肺脾气虚证

临床表现：气短，倦怠乏力，纳差呕恶，痞满，大便无力，便溏不爽。舌淡胖，苔白腻。

推荐处方：法半夏 9 g、陈皮 10 g、党参 15 g、炙黄芪 30 g、炒白术 10 g、茯苓 15 g、藿香 10 g、砂仁 6 g（后下）、甘草 6 g。

服法：每日 1 剂，水煎 400 mL，分 2 次服用，早晚各 1 次。

※ 气阴两虚证

临床表现：乏力，气短，口干，口渴，心悸，汗多，纳差，低热或不热，干咳少痰。舌干少津，脉细或虚无力。

推荐处方：南北沙参各 10 g、麦冬 15 g、西洋参 6 g，五味子 6 g、生石膏 15 g、淡竹叶 10 g、桑叶 10 g、芦根 15 g、丹参 15 g、生甘草 6 g。

服法：每日 1 剂，水煎 400 mL，分 2 次服用，早晚各 1 次。

十一、出院标准和出院后注意事项

（一）出院标准

1. 体温恢复正常 3 天以上。

2. 呼吸道症状明显好转。

3. 肺部影像学显示急性渗出性病变明显改善。

4. 连续两次痰、鼻咽拭子等呼吸道标本核酸检测阴性（采样时间至少间隔 24 小时）。

满足以上条件者可出院。

（二）出院后注意事项

1.定点医院要做好与患者居住地基层医疗机构间的联系，共享病历资料，及时将出院患者信息推送至患者辖区或居住地居委会和基层医疗卫生机构。

2.患者出院后，建议应继续进行 14 天的隔离管理和健康状况监测，佩戴口罩，有条件的居住在通风良好的单人房间，减少与家人的近距离密切接触，分餐饮食，做好手卫生，避免外出活动。

3.建议在出院后第二周和第四周到医院随访、复诊。

十二、转运原则

按照国家卫生健康委印发的《新型冠状病毒感染的肺炎病例转运工作方案（试行）》执行。

十三、医疗机构内感染预防与控制

严格按照国家卫健委《医疗机构内新型冠状病毒感染预防与控制技术指南（第一版）》《新型冠状病毒感染的肺炎防护中常见医用防护用品使用范围指引（试行）》的要求执行。

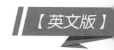

COVID-19 Pulmonary CT Features and Evolution

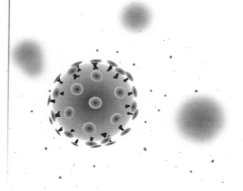

1

Introduction of COVID-19

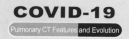
1.1 Discovery and Development History of COVID-19

On January 7, 2020, a new type of coronavirus was detected in the laboratory, and the whole genome sequence of the virus was obtained. A total of 15 positive cases of the new type of coronavirus were detected by the nucleic acid detection method. The virus was isolated from the sample of one positive patient, with typical coronavirus morphology under an electron microscope. On the same day, the expert group believed that the causative agent of the unidentified viral pneumonia case in Wuhan was preliminarily determined to be a novel coronavirus.

On January 20, 2020, the National Health Commission of the People's Republic of China(the abbreviation is China's National Health Commission) issued the Announcement No.1 of 2020, which included pneumonia with new coronavirus infection into the Class B infectious diseases stipulated in *the Law of the People's Republic of China on the Prevention and Treatment of Infectious Diseases*, and adopted the prevention and control measures for category infectious diseases. Pneumonia with new coronavirus infection shall be included in the management of quarantinable infectious diseases stipulated in *the Frontier Health and Quarantine Law of the People's Republic of China*.

On December 31, 2019, China reported a group of pneumonia cases in Wuhan, Hubei province, which resulted in the confirmation of a novel coronavirus.

On January 11, 2020, the first fatality occurred in Wuhan, who had been continuously exposed to seafood markets in southern China and was hospitalized after seven days of fever, cough and breathing difficulties.

On February 7, 2020, the National Health Commission issued a notice, deciding to temporarily name "Novel Coronavirus Pneumonia (NCP)".

On February 22, 2020, the official website of the National Health Commission issued a notice on the revision of the English name of the novel coronavirus pneumonia, deciding to change the English name of the novel coronavirus pneumonia to "COVID-19", in line with the name of the World Health Organization.

On 31 January 2020, the World Health Organization recommended that the current novel Coronavirus pneumonia be tentatively named "2019-nCoV acute respiratory disease" and the virus be tentatively named "2019-nCoV". "2019" stands for "the first year of emergence", "n" for "novel" and "CoV" for "Coronavirus".

On February 11, 2020, the Director-General of the World Health Organization Tedros Adhanorm Ghebreyesus announced in Geneva, Switzerland, the new coronavirus pneumonia was named "COVID-19", in which "CO" stands for "corona", "VI" for "virus" and "D" for "disease". On the same day, the International Commission on Taxonomy of Viruses named the new coronavirus SARS-CoV-2. Writing in a preprint on bioRxiv, ICTV's coronavirus research team highlighted the similarity between the new virus and SARS.

At 6 o'clock on April 14 2020, the cumulative number of confirmed cases of COVID-19 globally has exceeded 1.9 million, bringing the total number of confirmed cases to 1 912 923 and the cumulative number of deaths to 119 212. More than 580 000 cases have been confirmed in the United States, with 583 870 cases and 23 485 deaths. A total of 169 628 cases have been confirmed in Spain, with 17 628 deaths. A total of 159 516 cases have been confirmed in Italy, with 20 465 deaths. Outside the US, France, the UK, and Turkey all had more than 4000 new cases in a single day, with the largest number of new confirmed cases.

On March 8, 2020, a total of 25 561 cases were confirmed overseas, of which 2730 were cured and 501 died. The number of cases under treatment overseas (22 330) has surpassed that of China (20 611) and is growing rapidly.

2020 0306

2020 0308

2020 0319

2020 0414

On March 6, 2020, there was an outbreak of the novel coronavirus (COVID-19) in Europe. According to a report by the *European Times of France*, as of 20 o'clock on March 5 in Paris, a total of 5843 new coronavirus infections have been reported in Europe, an increase of 1347 cases compared with 8 o'clock on March 5 of these, Italy increased by 769 to 3858, Germany by 169 to 547 and France by 138 to 423.

By 19 March 2020, the death toll in Italy had surpassed that in China, with 41 035 cases of infection. The number of infections in the United States has also risen to more than 10 000.

1.2　Epidemiology of COVID-19

1.2.1　The Concept of Coronavirus

Coronavirus belongs to genera Beta-coronavirus under the Coronaviridae family. Coronavirus are enveloped, single-stranded RNA viruses, which are widely found in nature. At the same time, it is also an important pathogen of livestock, pets and even human diseases, and can cause a variety of acute and chronic diseases. Respiratory infection is one of the major effects of coronavirus on humans.

Since coronaviruses are sensitive to temperature, they grow well at 33 ℃ but are inhibited at 35 ℃ . Therefore, winter and early spring are the epidemic seasons for this virus disease. At the same time, coronavirus is also one of the main pathogens of the common cold in adults, and the infection rate in children is relatively high, mainly upper respiratory tract infection, which rarely affects the lower respiratory tract. In addition, the virus can also cause acute gastroenteritis in infants, the main symptoms are watery stool, fever, vomiting, and even blood watery stool in severe cases, very few cases can also cause nervous system syndrome.

2019-nCoV is the seventh known coronavirus to infect humans. The remaining six are HCoV-229E, HCoV-OC43, HCoV-NL63, HCoV-HKU1, SARS-CoV (causing Severe Acute Respiratory Syndrome) and MERS-CoV (causing Middle East Respiratory Syndrome). 2019-nCoV is a new pathogen, which is highly contagious and spreads quickly. It is neither influenza nor SARS.

1.2.2　Epidemic Status of COVID-19

By 24 : 00 on February 21, 2020, China's 31 provinces (autonomous regions, municipalities directly under the central government) and

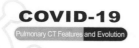

Xinjiang production and construction corps reported a total of 53 284 confirmed cases (in which 11 477 severe cases), 20 659 cases cured and discharged, 2345 cases dead , 76 288 cases confirmed and 5365 cases suspected cases. A total of 618 915 close contacts have been traced, and 113 564 remain under medical observation. In Hubei province, 13 557 cases have been cured and discharged from hospital (7206 in Wuhan), 2250 deaths (1774 in Wuhan) and 63 454 confirmed cases (45 660 in Wuhan).

By February 21, 2020, 100 new cases of crown pneumonia had been confirmed in South Korea, and a total of 204 cases had been confirmed 728 cases, the cumulative number of confirmed cases in Japan is 728, including 3 deaths; The Centers for Disease Control and Prevention (CDC) confirmed 34 new cases of COVID-19 in the United States.

As of 30 March 2020, the Ministry of Health in Spanish has confirmed 12 298 medical workers tested positive for novel coronavirus. On the same day, the National Institutes of Higher Health released data showing that the number of cases of novel Coronavirus among medical workers in Italy was 8 358, an increase of 595 from the previous day, and 63 physicians died from novel coronavirus.

Up to 11 : 00 Beijing time on March 20, 2020, there are 244 421 confirmed cases of COVID-19 worldwide, with 10 027 deaths and over 10 000 deaths. Nearly three months after the outbreak, almost 250 000 people worldwide have been infected with novel Coronavirus, which has spread to all continents except Antarctica. As the epidemic draws to a close in China, the situation in Europe, Iran, and the United States are getting worse, with the number of confirmed cases in seven countries topping 10 000.

As of 12 : 00 on 31 March 2020, 202 countries around the world have been hit by outbreaks of COVID-19. In addition to China, a total of 778 465 cases have been confirmed, 162 717 have been cured and 37 185 have died (involving 126 countries, of which the top 10 countries are Italy, Spain, the United States, France, Iran, the United Kingdom, the Netherlands, Germany, Belgium and Switzerland).

1.2.3 Infection Mechanism of COVID-19

On January 10, 2020, the data of the first genome sequence of a novel coronavirus from Wuhan was released. Later, the genome sequences of several novel Coronavirus isolated from patients were successively released. Institute Pasteur of Shanghai, Chinese Academy of Sciences, Pharmaceutical Engineering Technology Research Center for National Emergency Prevention and Control, Academy of Military Medicine and Center for Excellence in Molecular Plant Sciences, Chinese Academy of Sciences compared the novel coronavirus genome of Wuhan with the SARS-CoV and MERS-CoV, and found that there were 70% and 40% sequence similarity on average, Among them, the *spike* gene (encoding S-protein) of different coronaviruses interacting with host cells has greater differences (Fig. 1-2-1).

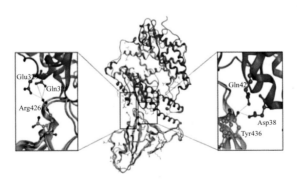

Fig. 1-2-1   The predictive structure and electron microscopy of novel coronavirus

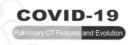
1.2.4 Animal-derived and COVID-19

In addition to its own characteristic changes, the coronavirus can also change with the transfer of the host. With the expansion of human activities, some viruses isolated from human beings spread to humans through wild animals. For example, the SARS virus in 2003 may have originated in bats and passed to humans through civet cats, its intermediate host. Therefore, finding the animal origin of the virus is crucial to understanding and controlling the spread of the virus.

The current cases of COVID-19 were first diagnosed in Wuhan. The researchers isolated and sequenced the genomes of nine hospitalized patients, eight of whom had traveled to the South China Seafood Market in Wuhan, and found that the genomes were about 88% consistent with the sequences of bat-SL-CovzC45 and bat-SL-CovXC21, two bat-derived coronaviruses found in Zhoushan, eastern China, in 2018. The team of Zhengli Shi from Wuhan Institute of Virology, Chinese Academy of Sciences, found that the sequence identity between 2019-nCoV and a bat coronavirus is as high as 96%. By comparing the seven conserved non-structural proteins, it was found that 2019-nCoV belongs to SARS-CoV, and the receptor of COVID-19 entering cells was ACE2, just like SARS-CoV. In February 2020, a new study by the research teams including Professor Yongyi Shen's of Guangdong Laboratory of Lingnan Modern Agricultural Science and Technology, South China Agricultural University showed that pangolin is a potential intermediate host of novel coronavirus. But so far there is no definite intermediate host.

1.2.5 Epidemic Characteristics of COVID-19

Novel coronavirus is mainly transmitted by respiratory droplets and contact, fecal-oral transmission is yet to be studied, and aerosol transmission may exist in medical institutions. After the virus is introduced into an area, without intervention, it will easily cause the occurrence of local cluster cases. However, strict isolation and increasing social distance and other control measures can effectively reduce the incidence of the virus. Almost everyone is susceptible to the novel coronavirus. Whether humans have immunity after infection needs further study. According to the research of Academician Nanshan Zhong, from the the analysis of confirmed and suspected cases, most of the patients are aged from 30 to 65 years old, among which 56 years old is the most, and the prevalence rate of people aged 18 years and below is relatively low (accounting for 2.4% of all reported cases). Most cases of children were found by tracing close contacts of adult patients' families, but no cases of transmission from children to adults were found; the age distribution of confirmed and suspected cases was similar; the proportion of truly asymptomatic infections is unclear, but it is relatively rare and is not a major factor in transmission. In terms of geographical analysis, the age of onset was younger in cities outside Wuhan. The incidence in males (37%) and females (27%) was significantly different per 100 000 population ($P < 0.001$), with an average latency of 4.75 (interquartile spacing 3.0 to 7.2) days. Compared with SARS-CoV, novel coronavirus has stronger transmission and lower fatality rate. Based on monitoring data at the individual level, early detection and treatment of elderly patients, especially elder men, is important.

1.3　Etiological Detection Value of COVID-19

According to the *Diagnosis and Treatment Protocol for COVID-19 (Trial Version 7)* released by the National Health Commission, real-

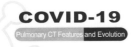

time fluorescent RT-PCR and viral genome sequencing are used as detection methods for etiology. Real-time fluorescent RT-PCR is one of the most direct and effective methods to detect the presence of viral nucleic acid in the blood and diagnose the presence or absence of pathogen infection. And reverse transcription-polymerase chain reaction (RT-PCR) is the most common technique for nucleic acid detection due to its technical sensitivity and wide application. However, some patients are clinically COVID-19, but the nucleic acid test results are negative. The possible reasons for this false negative clinical diagnosis are as follows: Firstly, the specificity, sensitivity, and stability of the kit need to be further optimized and verified, and the quality of the kit also needs to be improved. Secondly, the virus content at the sampling site and in the samples may affect the test results.

Currently, the most commonly used method is to collect nasopharyngeal swab. However, the randomness of the nasopharyngeal swab collection is relatively high, and the extraction of viral nucleic acid samples after sampling may be affected by individual differences. Moreover, the amount of virus in the upper respiratory tract, including the nasopharynx, maybe too small to meet the detection limits of the kit in the early stages of the disease. In addition, the storage and transportation of samples are also critical. Samples may be improperly preserved, which may affect the the extraction rate and quality of viral nucleic acid extraction, and affect the subsequent quantitative analysis.

1.4   CT Detection Value of COVID-19

With the deepening understanding of the COVID-19, the characteristic CT image changes and dynamic evolution of the disease become clearer. Due to its high resolution, CT has a high diagnostic sensitivity for novel coronavirus pneumonia, which is of great significance for early diagnosis, early isolation, early treatment and reduction of transmission, thus shortening the duration of the epidemic Therefore, lung CT plays an increasingly important role in the diagnosis and judgment of novel coronavirus pneumonia. Among the diagnostic criteria for COVID-19 patients in the *Diagnosis and Treatment Protocol for COVID-19 (Trial Version 7)* released by the National Health Commission, CT imaging features of COVID-19 are an important condition for the diagnosis of suspected cases.

2

Clinical Manifestations and Treatment of COVID-19

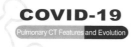

2.1 Clinical Classification of COVID-19

According to the *Diagnosis and Treatment Protocol for COVID-19 (Trial Version 7)* released by the National Health Commission, the clinical types of COVID-19 can be classified into mild, moderate, severe and critical.

2.1.1 Mild Type

The patient had symptoms of fever and respiratory tract, and the manifestations of pneumonia could be seen on imaging.

2.1.2 Moderate Type

The patient with fever, respiratory tract, and other symptoms, lung CT can be seen pneumonia. Most patients presented with fever, dry cough and fatigue, while a few presented with pharyngeal pain, nasal congestion, nausea, diarrhea, chest tightness, decreased appetite, muscle soreness, dizziness, headache, etc., with no specificity. Chest imaging showed pneumonia.

2.1.3 Severe Type

Adult patients met any of the following criteria: ①Onset of shortness of breath, respiratory rate（RR）$\geqslant$ 30 times/min; ②At rest, saturation $\leqslant$ 93%; ③Arterial partial blood oxygen pressure (PaO_2)/fraction of inspiration oxygen (FiO_2) $\leqslant$ 300 mmHg (1 mmHg=0.133 kPa), high altitude (above 1000 m) should be corrected according to the formula (PaO_2/FiO_2) × [atmospheric pressure (mmHg) /760]; ④Lung imaging showed significant progression of > 50% within 24-48 hours.

Elderly people with severe basic diseases are more likely to develop into critical type.

2.1.4　Heavy and Critical type

Adult patients meet any of the following criteria: ①Respiratory failure and need mechanical ventilation; ②Go into shock; ③Patients with other organ failure should be monitored in ICU.

2.2　Clinical Manifestations of COVID-19

According to the current epidemiological investigation, the incubation period of COVID-19 is 1 to 14 days, mostly 3 to 7 days, but it has been reported as long as 24 days.

2.2.1　Mild Type

The clinical manifestations of the patients were only mild respiratory symptoms such as low fever, fatigue, dry cough, and some patients even had no clinical symptoms, and chest imaging showed no signs of pneumonia.

2.2.2　Moderate Type

Most of the patients presented with fever, dry cough, and fatigue, while a few presented with pharyngeal pain, nasal congestion, diarrhea, chest tightness, loss of appetite, muscle aches, dizziness, headache, etc., with was no specificity. Chest imaging showed pneumonia.

2.2.3　Heavy and Critical Type

One week after the onset of the disease, generally lasts for 7 to 14 days, the patients may have dyspnea and/or hypoxemia. Chest tightness, cough, fatigue, decreased appetite, dizziness and other symptoms are more likely to occur in patients with moderate type. The body temperature of patients with this type may be moderate to low fever, or even no obvious fever. Severe cases develop into acute

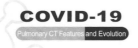
respiratory distress syndrome, septic shock, refractory metabolic acidosis, severe coagulation dysfunction, and multiple organ failure within days or even hours.

2.3 Characteristics of Laboratory Tests of COVID-19

In the early stage of the disease, the total number of white blood cells in the peripheral blood of the patients was normal or decreased. In the case of bacterial infection, the total number of white cells could be increased, and the absolute value of lymphocytes decreased, mainly the decrease of CD4$^+$T cells and CD8$^+$T cells. In a small number of patients, the number of platelets decreased, while in some patients, liver enzymes, creatinine dehydrogenase, creatine kinase and prothrombin decreased. C-reactive protein and erythrocyte sedimentation rate increased in most patients, and procalcitonin and troponin were basically normal. In severe cases, peripheral blood lymphocytes progressively decreased and d-dimer increased. The inflammatory factors IL-6 and IL-10 increased in most severe and critical patients but decreased rapidly with the improvement of the disease.

The nucleic acid of the novel coronavirus can be detected in nasopharyngeal swabs, sputum, alveolar lavage fluid, blood, stool, and other specimens. Pharyngeal swabs are prone to false negatives. In order to improve the positive rate of nucleic acid test, we recommend that sputum specimens should be collected and sent for testing as soon as possible.

2.4　Diagnostic Criteria of COVID-19

2.4.1　Suspected Case

Clinical manifestations: ① Fever and/or respiratory symptoms; ② Typical imaging manifestations of COVID-19; ③ Early white blood cell count was normal or decreased, lymphocyte count decreased. Meet any 2 or 3 of the clinical manifestations, and have an epidemiological history.

2.4.2　Confirmed Case

The suspected case has one of the following etiological evidence: ① Novel coronavirus nucleic acid was tested positive by RT-PCR; ② Viral gene sequencing is highly homologous with the novel coronavirus; ③ Novel coronavirus-specific IgG antibody and IgG antibody were positive, and the serum novel coronavirus IgG antibody was increased 4 times or more from negative in the recovery period than in the acute phase.

2.5　Treatment of COVID-19

2.5.1　Treatment Plan

1. Closely monitor the changes in patients' vital signs: body temperature, respiratory rhythm, frequency, depth, and blood oxygen saturation.

2. Patients with oxygen therapy could adjust oxygen flow according to their blood oxygen saturation and apply high-flow nasal cannula oxygen therapy (HFNCOT) as necessary.

3. Adjust the inspiratory pressure, expiratory pressure and oxygen concentration and other parameters according to the patient's tidal volume and oxygenation index.

4. For patients undergoing endotracheal intubation or tracheotomy,

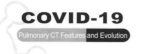
closed type sputum aspiration and artificial airway management should be adopted under three-level protective measures.

2.5.2 Observation of Disease

1. Closely observe the patient's consciousness and general state, such as cough, chest tightness, muscle ache, fatigue, diarrhea, appetite, etc., and pay attention to whether the symptoms are aggravated or new symptoms appear.

2. Strengthen the monitoring and treatment of patients' basic diseases, such as hypertension, diabetes, chronic renal insufficiency, etc.

3. Prevention and timely treatment of complications.

2.5.3 Drug Therapy

2.5.3.1 Mild Type

Bed rest, nutritional support, and adequate calories. COVID-19 is lack of clear and effective antiviral drugs, so alpha interferon (5 million units per time + 2 mL sterile water injection for adults, atomization and absorption, b.i.d), lopinavir/ritonavir (500 mg per time for adult, b.i.d), abby dole (200 mg per time for adult, t.i.d), phosphorus acid chloroquine (500 mg per time for adult, b.i.d), etc., can only be chosen at this stage. But we need to pay attention to the antiviral drug adverse reactions, such as nausea, diarrhea, etc., and don't recommend the simultaneous use of three or more antiviral drugs.

2.5.3.2 Moderate Type

General treatment with light, closely monitor patients with symptoms and signs, such as continuous high fever, difficulty breathing, oxygen desaturation, and so on. In case of persistent high fever, difficulty in breathing or oxygen saturation, nasal catheter should be used for oxygen inhalation. Antiviral therapy can be tried: alpha interferon

(5 million units per time + 2 mL sterile water injection for adults, atomization and absorption, b.i.d), lopinavir/ritonavir (500 mg per time for adult, b.i.d), abby dole (200 mg per time for adult, t.i.d), phosphorus acid chloroquine (500 mg per time for adult, b.i.d), etc.. When oxygenation index is less than 300, immediately follow the heavy standard.

2.5.3.3 Severe Type

Principles of treatment: on the basis of symptomatic treatment, actively treat complications, treat basic diseases, prevent secondary infection, and provide timely organ function support. Nasal catheters are used for oxygen inhalation, if necessary, through high nasal flow and non-invasive ventilator ventilation. Routine non-invasive positive pressure ventilation is not recommended for patients who fail to treat HFNCOT. We have the following suggestions.

1. Continuous monitoring of blood oxygen saturation, blood gas analysis, regular review of chest CT.

2. Antiviral treatment: alpha interferon (5 million units per time + 2 mL sterile water injection for adults, atomization and absorption, b.i.d), lopinavir/ritonavir (500 mg per time for adult, b.i.d), abby dole (200 mg per time for adult, t.i.d), phosphorus acid chloroquine (500 mg per time for adult, b.i.d), etc.

3. When early diagnosis is severe, low-dose glucocorticoid treatment should be given immediately [mepredonal 0.5-1 mg / (kg·d), gradually decreasing to discontinuance according to the improvement of symptoms and blood oxygen saturation, with a course of 3-10 days].

4. Can be combined with human immunoglobulin.

5. Routine prophylactic use of antibiotics is not recommended,with signs of infection (such as elevated white blood cells), intravenous

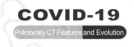

antibiotics.

6.Regulate intestinal microecology and other supportive treatments.

2.5.3.4 Critical Type

Invasive mechanical ventilation: ARDS severity shall be determined by positive end expiratory pressure (PEEP) to reduce the lung injury like expiratory machine (4-6 mL/kg) and low inspiratory pressure (platform pressure $<$ 30 cmH$_2$O). If necessary, consider extracorporeal membrane oxygenation (ECMO) therapy. We have the following suggestions.

1. Closely monitor blood gas analysis and bedside chest X-ray.

2. Methylprednisolone 80-160 mg/d was reduced step by step until discontinuation according to the improvement of symptoms and oxygen saturation.

3. Antiviral therapy: Alpha interferon (5 million units per time + 2 mL sterile water injection for adults, twice a day for atomization and absorption), lopinavir/ritonavir (500 mg per time for adult, b.i.d), abby dole (200 mg per time for adult, b.i.d), phosphorus acid chloroquine (500 mg per time for adult, b.i.d), etc., can be chosen for the treatment of COVID-19.

4. Can be combined with human immunoglobulin.

5. If there are signs of infection (e.g. elevated white blood cells), intravenous antibiotics should be used.

6. Regulate intestinal microecology and other supportive treatments.

7. Artificial liver treatment.

8. The convalescent were treated with plasma.

9. Immunotherapy: tocilizumab therapy can be tried for the patient with increased IL-6 levels.

10. Treatment for combination with shock: ①fluid resuscitation, normal saline and equilibrium solution can be selected, and human serum albumin can be supplemented if necessary; ②Vasoactive drugs, norepinephrine is recommended as the first choice of vasoactive drugs, other options can be dopamine, pituitrin, etc.

2.5.4　Psychological Assessment and Support

1. Evaluate the patients' cognitive change, emotional response, and behavioral change, and give psychological adjustment and other intervention measures.

2. Provide appropriate emotional support and encourage the patient to build up confidence in overcoming the disease.

3. Provide continuous correct information support to eliminate uncertainty and anxiety.

4. Give good health guidance to patients to ensure adequate sleep and a good psychological state.

2.5.5　Nutritional Support

1. Strengthen nutrition support, give high caloric high protein high vitamin digestible diet.

2. Enteral or parenteral nutrition support should be given to severe patients and energy supply should be 25-35 kcal/(kg·d). Enteral nutrition should be started as soon as possible and prevent reflux aspiration.

2.5.6　Respiratory Rehabilitation Exercise

Choose appropriate respiratory rehabilitation exercises, such as airway clearance training, breathing exercises, lip contraction breathing,

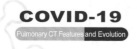
abdominal breathing, etc.

2.5.7　TCM Syndrome Differentiation and Treatment

COVID-19 can be divided into early, middle, critical and recovery stages. In the early stage, the lung was depressed by cold and humidity and the external cold and internal heat in the middle stage, the lung was mixed with cold and heat in the severe stage, there was internal closure of epidemic virus in the lung; in the convalescent stage there was deficiency of the spleen-energy and lung-energy. According to the stages, classification of syndrome differentiation and treatment, the combined therapy of cooling with warming was using through the whole process of treatment.

2.6　Discharge Criteria and Follow-up for COVID-19

The body temperature returned to normal for more than 3 days, respiratory symptoms were significantly improved, the lesions in the lungs were significantly absorbed, and the respiratory pathogens nucleic acid test was negative for 2 consecutive times (sampling interval was at least 1 day). In view of the recent occurrence of nucleic acid positive detection in feces, we included negative detection of fecal pathogen nucleic acid in the discharge standard.

After discharge, patients were isolated at home for 14 days and followed up in the outpatient department after 2 weeks, 1 month, 3 months, 6 months and 1 year. Blood routine, blood biochemistry, blood oxygen saturation, lung CT and lung function should be rechecked during the follow-up visit. If necessary, novel coronavirus pathogen test should be performed.

3

Procedures and Diagnostic Specification for COVID-19

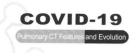
The situation of COVID-19 pneumonia prevention and control is grim. Imaging examination, as an important link in the diagnosis of COVID-19 pneumonia, plays an important role in screening, diagnosis, prediction and prognosis of COVID-19. At present, pulmonary CT is an important means of early diagnosis, and radiographers are in the front line of epidemic prevention and control. Faced with the double responsibility and pressure of infection prevention and control and radiation protection, it is particularly important to standardize imaging examination process. With reference to the *Protocol on Prevention and Control of COVID-19 (Version 6)* printed and distributed by National Health Committee and *Novel Coronavirus (2019-nCoV) Radiological Examination Protocol and Expert Consensus on Infection Prevention and Control (Version 1)* released by Imaging Technology Branch of Chinese Medical Association, and based on practical work experience, different imaging examination equipment and different examination procedures were developed according to different patients' physical conditions.

3.1 Procedures for Testing COVID-19

In order to better prevent and control the epidemic situation and prevent cross-infection, we should try our best to create conditions to set up an independent medical imaging examination area or special radiological examination equipment, and arrange special personnel to carry out imaging examination of patients with fever.

3.1.1 Special Areas and Special Machines

Pollution areas, potential pollution areas and clean areas should be strictly divided, and work in their respective areas in strict accordance with the prevention and control requirements. No pollution should be caused by illegally crossing or confusing the boundaries of the zones. We encourage qualified hospitals to set up separate CT room and digital X-ray imaging system (DR) room, and equipped with an independent waiting area for receiving the above-mentioned patients with fever. On the choice of the machine room, the machine room with an independent operation room should be selected, and the operation room should not be shared with other machines. If the above conditions cannot be met, the machine room and the operation room shall be sterilized in strict accordance with the disinfection process after inspection, and the air disinfection shall be carried out in other machine rooms connected with the operation room. Ordinary patients will seek treatment in designated areas to reduce the possibility of contact with suspected and confirmed patients and to reduce the risk of nosocomial or iatrogenic infection.

3.1.2 Specialized Personnel

Reasonable arrangement of personnel within the machine section, shall be fixed personnel placement for the patients with fever accepts work, need to live and work in the area of the hospital dedicated isolation, one work cycle after the access to the special area for medical observation, observation period after the detection of nucleic acid and lung CT, check without exception can resume normal life, back to work.

Within the department, personnel should be reasonably arranged, and specialized personnel should be assigned to receive the above-mentioned patients with fever, and need to live and work in the area of the hospital dedicated isolation. At the end of one working cycle, the patient entered the special isolation zone for medical observation. After the observation period, nucleic acid and lung CT were detected. If

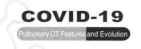
there is no abnormality, they can return to normal life and work.People who have direct close contact with patients with fever, suspected or confirmed COVID-19 are at high risk of occupational exposure. Attention should be paid to isolation and protection to minimize the risk of nosocomial infection among medical staff. Medical personnel entering the room delicated to fever must prepare according to the secondary protection standards: work clothes plus disposable isolation clothing or protective clothing, N95 mask, goggles or disposable eye screen, disposable hats, single layer latex gloves. The rest of the medical staff in the machine room should strictly implement the primary protection. At the same time, the department should emphasize the importance of hand hygiene, medical staff should consciously implement the work of hand hygiene, to protect patients, but also to protect themselves.

3.1.3 Level of Infection Prevention and Control in Radiological Diagnostic Examination

3.1.3.1 General Protection

It is applicable to the staff far away from patients in the radiological diagnosis room, post-processing room and information management room. Wear disposable work caps, disposable surgical masks.

3.1.3.2 Primary Prevention

It is applicable to the staff in the areas of pre-triage, registration, tablet collection, general radiology examination room, etc. Wear disposable work caps, disposable surgical masks (type N95 or above medical protective masks for contact with patients with epidemiological history), work clothes (wear isolation clothes for contact with patients with epidemiological history), disposable latex gloves when necessary, and strictly carry out hand hygiene.

3.1.3.3　Secondary Prevention

It is suitable for the close operators to perform radiological examination for suspected and confirmed COVID-19 patients in fever out-patient department, infection out-patient department, respiratory out-patient department, isolation ward, special radiological examination room, and other places to conduct the radiological examination on suspected and confirmed patients. Wear disposable work caps, type N95 or above medical protective masks, goggles or protective face screens, disposable latex gloves, medical protective clothing (with protective clothing in the isolation ward), disposable shoe covers or boot covers, and strictly carry out hand hygiene.

3.1.3.4　Tertiary Prevention

It is suitable for close operator to perform radiological examination for suspected or confirmed severe COVID-19 patients in relatively closed environments and prolonged exposure to high concentrations of aerosols. On the basis of secondary protection, wear protective face screen, goggles, comprehensive respiratory protective device or positive pressure type head cover, and strictly carry out hand hygiene.

The level of infection prevention and control should be based on the type of patient exposed and the degree of exposure to the patient, and should not be limited to the specific places mentioned above.

3.1.3.5　Wear and Remove Protective Clothing

1. Procedures for wearing protective equipment:seven steps to wash hands→wear a hat→wear a medical protective mask (N95, air leakage test)→wear protective clothing (after removing shoes) → wear latex gloves (inner layer) → wear disposable isolation clothing→wear latex gloves (outer layer)→wear rubber boots→wear boots→wear goggles or protective face screen-check the tightness of

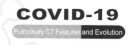
wearing.

2. Process of removing protective equipment

(1) contaminated area: remove visible dirt→ hand hygiene→ remove outer shoe cover→ hand hygiene→ remove isolation clothing together with outer gloves→ hand hygiene.

(2) Semi-contaminated area: remove goggles or protective face screen→ hand hygiene→ remove protective clothing with inner gloves and boot covers→ hand hygiene→ remove medical protective mask (N95)→ remove hat→ wash hands in 7 steps.

3.1.3.6 Standard for Terminal Disinfection of Radiology Room

1. Wipe and sterilize all surfaces and equipment with with 75% alcohol or 1000 mg/L chlorine-containing disinfectant and wipe with clean water after 30 minutes.

2. Air disinfection: the circulatory air disinfecting machine can be used for continuous disinfection, or ultraviolet irradiation can be used for continuous disinfection without human being for 30 minutes each time.

3. Clean the floor with 500 mg/L chlorine-containing disinfectant and clean with water after 30 minutes.

4. All garbage shall be tied with gooseneck and placed in the designated area. All waste from patients shall be treated as infectious medical waste and shall be managed strictly in accordance with the *Regulations on the Management of Medical Waste and Measures for the Management of Medical Waste in Medical and Health Istitutions.*

3.2 Procedures for Patients with Fever (with Epidemiological History), Suspected and Confirmed COVID-19

3.2.1 The Technician's Preparation before Examination

In order to maximize the protection of medical staff in the department, we recommend that both DR and CT be performed by the same technician. Before the operation, the technician should strictly implement secondary prevention. If sputum aspiration, respiratory tract sampling, endotracheal intubation and tracheotomy are likely to occur, the patient must perform tertiary prevention, when respiratory secretions and substances in the body are sprayed or sputtered.

3.2.2 The Patient's Preparation before Examination

Before examination, the nurse on duty should contact contact the radiology department in advance and inform the radiologist of the patient's situation, and then wait for the radiologist to open the entrance door of the patient's special channel. Patients should wear surgical masks or N95 masks throughout the examination. According to the examination site, remove metal ornaments and other high-density items (such as necklaces, earrings, and clothes with metal zippers) shall be removed in advance. Patients who can move independently will be accompanied to the examination room for inspection after the nurse conducts propaganda work. For patients who need to be transported by cart or bed, the nurse escorts the patient to the examination room for examination after strict hand disinfection. The personnel of the security department should coordinate with the escort to evacuate the medical staff, and advise the medical staff to

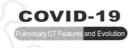

keep a distance of more than 1.5 m and go to the special channel. They should avoid contact with the surrounding environment and pedestrians as far as possible. After the patient's bundle examination, they should be transported back to the isolation area, and the transportation tools should be timely disinfected.

3.2.3　Examination Process and Requirements

Before the examination, the technician should carefully check the application form and matters needing attention, clarify the purpose and requirements of the examination, ask the name of the patient, check the wristband of the patient, and do the work of "three checks and seven verifications". Do the radiation protection of the non-inspection site, and carry out respiratory training as required. Close communication with patients should be avoided as far as possible, in addition to positioning, patients should be kept at a distance of 1-1.5 m or more on the premise of ensuring patient safety. Conditions permitting, hospitals should make use of the machine's intelligent riser system for inspection.

If the patient's condition requires the injection of contrast agent for examination or other situations that require the nurse to have direct contact with the patient, the nurse should perform secondary prevention as required.

3.2.4　Disinfection after Examination

After the patient has been examined, change the sheets and wipe and disinfect all equipment and surfaces that have been touched. For suspected or confirmed COVID-19 patients, air disinfection should be carried out immediately for 30 minutes with an air disinfecting machine. At the same time, 1000 mg/L chlorine-containing disinfectant should be used to mop the floor, and the floor should be cleaned again with clean water Put the contaminated disposable items into a double-layer medical waste bag, use a gooseneck sealed mouth, spray the outer surface of the bag with chlorine disinfection solution or 75% alcohol, and then put a yellow waste bag into the bag. After the gooseneck dressing, put a "COVID-19" label on the bag, contact the cleaning office, and have the medical waste sealed and transported by a designated person. In the machine room, wipe the desktop, door, door handle and all other items with 1000 mg/L of chlorine-containing disinfectant towels in order from low to high according to the possibility of contamination. After all procedures are completed, follow the seven-step washing technique to strictly implement hand hygiene.

(Note: when a suspected patient and a confirmed patient are seen at the same time, the suspected patient should be inspected first, then the confirmed patient, meanwhile the above mentioned disinfection should be strictly carried out between the two patients.)

3.3　Procedures for Common Fever and Common Patients (Suspected COVID-19 Found on Tests)

3.3.1　The Technician's Preparation before Examination

Prior to operation, the technician should strictly perform primary prevention. In case of sputum aspiration, respiratory tract sampling, endotracheal intubation, tracheotomy and other situations that are likely to cause the injection or spatter of respiratory secretions and substances in the patient, the technician should perform secondary prevention.

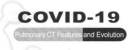

3.3.2 The Patient's Preparation before Examination

The patient should wear surgical masks or N95 masks throughout the examination without affecting the image quality. According to the inspection site, remove metal ornaments and other high density items (such as necklaces, earrings, clothing with metal zippers, etc.) from the site.

3.3.3 Examination Process and Requirements

Before the examination, the technician should carefully check the application form and matters needing attention,clarify the purpose and requirements of the examination, ask the name of the patient, check the wristband of the inpatient, and do the work of "three inspections and seven verifications". Do radiation protection on non-inspection sites and perform respiratory training as required.

3.3.4 Method of Examination

After examination, the image should be scanned carefully to assess whether there is a possibility of COVID-19. If there is a suspected tendency, immediately contact the diagnostic team physician for assistance in diagnosis. Meanwhile, patients are requested to wait in the machine room for the septum while the technician should change the personal protective equipment. If the patient is highly suspected by diagnostic physician as well, you should report to the on-site leader or senior physician, notify the fever clinic by telephone, and escort the patient out of the examination room. Then the remaining patients waiting outside the door of the machine room should be arranged to other machine rooms for inspection.

3.3.5 Disinfection after Examination

After the patient has been examined, change the sheets and wipe and disinfect all equipment and surfaces that have been touched. For suspected or confirmed COVID-19 patients, air disinfection should be carried out immediately for 30 minutes with an air disinfecting machine. At the same time, 1000 mg/L chlorine-containing disinfectant should be used to mop the floor, and the floor should be cleaned again with clean water put the contaminated disposable items into a double-layer medical waste bag, use a gooseneck sealed mouth, spray the outer surface of the bag with chlorine disinfection solution or 75% alcohol, and then put a yellow waste bag into the bag. After the gooseneck dressing, put a "COVID-19" label on the bag, contact the cleaning office, and have the medical waste sealed and transported by a designated person. In the machine room, wipe the desktop, door, door handle and all other items with 1000 mg/L of chlorine-containing disinfectant towels in order from low to high according to the possibility of contamination. After all procedures are completed, follow the seven-step washing technique to strictly implement hand hygiene. Manage every entrance into and out of the machine room, do not allow irrelevant personnel to enter.

3.4 Examination Procedures of Common Patients with Fever and Common Patients

3.4.1 The Technician's Preparation before Examination

Prior to operation, the technician should strictly perform the primary prevention. In case of sputum aspiration, respiratory tract sampling, endotracheal intubation and tracheotomy, which are likely to cause the injection or spatter of respiratory secretions and substances in the patient, the technician should perform secondary prevention (Fig.3-4-1).

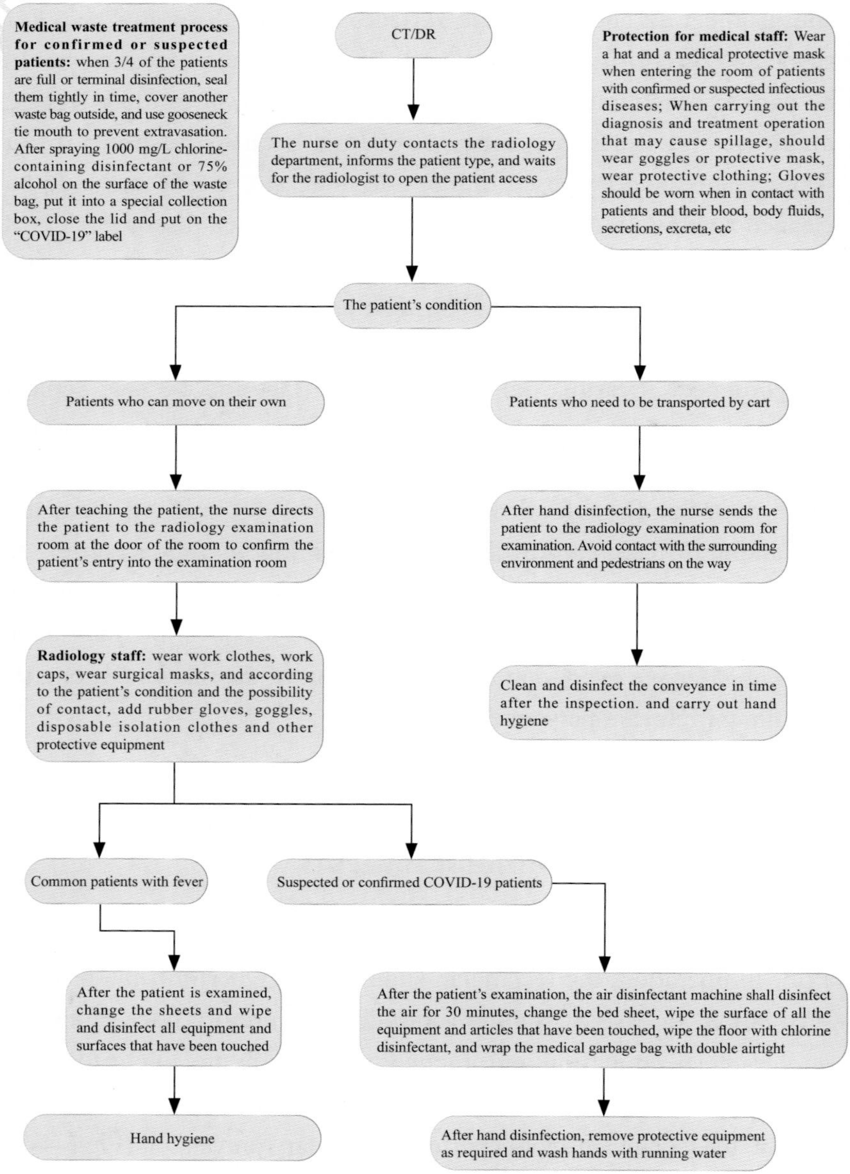

Medical waste treatment process for confirmed or suspected patients: when 3/4 of the patients are full or terminal disinfection, seal them tightly in time, cover another waste bag outside, and use gooseneck tie mouth to prevent extravasation. After spraying 1000 mg/L chlorine-containing disinfectant or 75% alcohol on the surface of the waste bag, put it into a special collection box, close the lid and put on the "COVID-19" label

CT/DR

Protection for medical staff: Wear a hat and a medical protective mask when entering the room of patients with confirmed or suspected infectious diseases; When carrying out the diagnosis and treatment operation that may cause spillage, should wear goggles or protective mask, wear protective clothing; Gloves should be worn when in contact with patients and their blood, body fluids, secretions, excreta, etc

The nurse on duty contacts the radiology department, informs the patient type, and waits for the radiologist to open the patient access

The patient's condition

Patients who can move on their own

Patients who need to be transported by cart

After teaching the patient, the nurse directs the patient to the radiology examination room at the door of the room to confirm the patient's entry into the examination room

After hand disinfection, the nurse sends the patient to the radiology examination room for examination. Avoid contact with the surrounding environment and pedestrians on the way

Radiology staff: wear work clothes, work caps, wear surgical masks, and according to the patient's condition and the possibility of contact, add rubber gloves, goggles, disposable isolation clothes and other protective equipment

Clean and disinfect the conveyance in time after the inspection. and carry out hand hygiene

Common patients with fever

Suspected or confirmed COVID-19 patients

After the patient is examined, change the sheets and wipe and disinfect all equipment and surfaces that have been touched

After the patient's examination, the air disinfectant machine shall disinfect the air for 30 minutes, change the bed sheet, wipe the surface of all the equipment and articles that have been touched, wipe the floor with chlorine disinfectant, and wrap the medical garbage bag with double airtight

Hand hygiene

After hand disinfection, remove protective equipment as required and wash hands with running water

Fig. 3-4-1　Fever patient(radiology) workflow

3.4.2   The Patient's Preparation before Examination

Patients should wear surgical masks or N95 masks throughout the examination without affecting the image quality. According to the inspection site, remove metal ornaments and other high-density items (such as necklaces, earrings, clothing with metal zippers, etc.) from the site.

3.4.3   Examination Procedures and Requirements

Before the examination, the technician should carefully check the application form and matters needing attention, clarify the purpose and requirements of the examination, ask the name of the patient, check the wristband of the inpatient, and do the work of "three checks and seven verifications". Do radiation protection on non-inspection sites and perform respiratory training as required.

3.4.4   Disinfection after Examination

Patients with common fever should be treated as emergency patients, and a report should be issued within half an hour. The general machine room should be disinfected twice a day, and the items and equipment surfaces in the machine room should be wiped with wipes that can reach a high level of disinfection. The personnel on duty and before going off duty in the afternoon should disinfect the equipment in their work areas once a time.

3.5   Procedures for Clinical Schemes of Patients with Fever (with an Epidemiological History), Suspected and Confirmed COVID-19

3.5.1   The technician's Preparation before Examination

The hospital should prepare a mobile DR as a special device to be

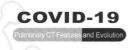
placed in the isolation ward for use by patients with fever (with an epidemiological history), suspected patients, and confirmed novel coronavirus patients. Prior to operation, the technician should strictly implement secondary prevention.In case of sputum aspiration, respiratory tract sampling, endotracheal intubation, tracheotomy and other situations that may occur in patients with respiratory secretions or spatter, the technician must perform tertiary prevention.

3.5.2 The Patient's Preparation before Examination

The patient should wear surgical masks or N95 masks throughout the examination without affecting the image quality. According to the inspection site, remove metal ornaments and other high density items (such as necklaces, earrings, clothing with metal zippers, etc.) from the site.

3.5.3 Examination Procedures and Requirements

Before the examination, the technician should carefully check the application form and matters needing attention, clarify the purpose and requirements of the examination, ask the name of the patient, check the wristband of the inpatient, and do the work of "three inspections and seven verifications". Do radiation protection on non-inspection sites and perform respiratory training as required. Close communication with patients should be avoided as far as possible, in addition to positioning, patients should be kept at a distance of 1-1.5 m or more on the premise of ensuring patient safety.

3.5.4 Disinfection after Examination

After the patient is examined, wipe and disinfect all equipment and surfaces that have been touched. Wash hands strictly by seven steps. As a close contact, the inspection technician should work in the isolation area for two weeks. After leaving the isolation ward, the patient entered the special isolation zone for medical observation, and at the end of the observation period nucleic acid and lung CT were detected. If there is no abnormality, they can return to normal life and work.

3.6　Screening Techniques of COVID-19

3.6.1　Digital Radiography (DR) Examination Scheme

3.6.1.1　Matters Needing Attention in Inspection

1. Configure a dedicated DR for COVID-19 patients.

2. Carry out equipment and room management in strict accordance with the above disinfection measures.

3. Bedside photography is recommended for critically ill patients.

3.6.1.2　Radiographic Screening Program for Adults

1. Photography distance: 180 cm.

2. Filter grid: minimum grid ratio 10 ∶ 1.

3. Exposure conditions: 125 kV, automatic exposure technology of ionization chamber.

4. Photographic position: posterior and anterior, with the center line aligned with the horizontal position of the sixth thoracic vertebra perpendicular to the incident position of the detector.

5. Protection requirements: cover the rest of your body as much as possible with lead aprons.

6. Breathing requirements: collect breath after a deep inhalation.

3.6.1.3　Screening Program for Patients Aged 0-3 Years and Above Who Do Not Cooperate

1. Photographic distance: 100 cm.

2. Filter grid: not used.

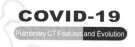
3. Exposure conditions: 50-60 kV, 0.6-2 mAs.

4. Photographic position: anterior and posterior, with the help of the patient's family members to fix the position,the center line is shot vertically into the center of the line between the two nipples.

5. Protection requirements: cover the rest of your body as much as possible with lead aprons.

3.6.1.4　Mobile Bedside X-ray Examination Program

1. Special mobile bedside X-ray machines are equipped in key areas such as the COVID-19 isolation wards to shoot for critically ill patients.

2. Before entering the isolation ward of COVID-19, the technician should strictly perform secondary protection. In case of any work that may occur such as sputum aspiration, respiratory sampling, endotracheal intubation and tracheotomy, which may cause the injection or spattering of respiratory secretions and substances in the patient, the technician must perform tertiary protection.

3. Take photos beside the bed, protect the plate detector or IP plate, and suggest to cover the plate with a plastic bag and sterilize it after use.

3.6.2　CT Examination Program

3.6.2.1　Matters Needing Attention for Examination

1. Designated CT room and specialized personnel should be arranged to check patients with fever, and the machine room should be an independent operation room, not Shared with other machines, and the waiting room should also be an independent space.

2. For patients diagnosed with novel coronavirus, a closed-loop examination process and path of "delivery→examination→return to the ward" was established under the coordination of the hospital infection office, medical office, radiology department, and ward.

3. Patients in the fever clinic enter the CT room through the designated channel, and return to the fever clinic through the original way after the examination.

4. After the scanning of confirmed patients is completed, the machine room should be sterilized according to the terminal disinfection standard of the radiology department.

5. After the CT operator completes the examination, the hand hygiene is performed.

6. If the machine room adopts the central air conditioning of the fresh air system, the air supply and exhaust volume of the air conditioning should be turned on to the maximum; if the machine room adopts ordinary central air conditioning is used in the machine room, the central air conditioning in the machine room and operation room should be shut down, and the standby independent air conditioning should be turned on. If there is no independent air conditioning, the central air conditioning should be turned on after inspection and disinfection.

7. The inspection bed should be covered with disposable sheets to avoid folding and cover the entire inspection bed;when using protective products, isolate the patient's body and clothing with disposable medium.

The inspection technician should pay attention to "three inspections and seven verifications", and make clear the purpose and requirements of the inspection. The patient and the accompanying personnel should wear the medical-surgical mask or N95 medical protective mask throughout the process of examination High-density items should be removed from the patient inspection area. Before the scan, the patients should be given breathing training. Generally, the breath should be held at the end of inhalation. The patients who cannot breathe properly will be ordered to breathe calmly and avoid cough.

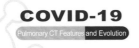
The inspection technician should try to use intercom when explaining the matters needing attention. For patients who are able to cooperate, the examination technician can guide the patient to position in the operation room by voice control on the premise of ensuring the patient's safety, or ask the attendant to assist the patient to get on the examination bed. When the examination technician is required to place himself/herself, keep a distance of more than 1 m from the patient as far as possible. If a distance of more than 1 m cannot be guaranteed, keep the head as far as possible from the respiratory tract of the patient. Wash hands with quick-drying hand sanitizer before and after contact with patients; The patient must wear a mask when entering the examination area and throughout the examination.

3.6.2.2 CT Scanning Program

1. Scanning body position: supine position is normally taken, and the head is held on both arms. For patients who have difficulty lifting their arms, place them at either side of the body.

2. Scanning method: spiral scanning.

3. Scanning range: for general patients, scan from the tip of the lung to the bottom of the diaphragm (including bilateral costal diaphragmatic angles). Patients with poor breath-holding should be scanned from the bottom of the diaphragm to the tip of the lung (the respiratory movement range at the bottom of the lung is greater than that at the tip of the lung) to reduce the artifacts of respiratory movement caused by poor breath-holding in the lower fields of both lungs and ensure image quality.

4. Scanning parameters: generally, spiral scanning is adopted, the voltage is 120 kV, intelligent radiation dose tracking technology (50-350 mAs) is used, and the thickness of the acquisition layer is 0.5-1.5 mm.

5. CT scan of children is performed at a low dose, and radiation

dose can be as low as 20 mAs.

3.6.2.3　CT Image Post-Processing

1. Post-processing of conventional images: lung window images (lung window: window width 1000-1500 Hu, window level -650--500 Hu) and mediastinal window images (mediastinal window: window width 250-300 Hu, window level 30-50 Hu) were reconstructed with 5mm thickness.

2. Post-processing of thin-layer image: build thin-layer lung window image with a thickness of layer less than 1 mm (lung window algorithm, window width 1000-1500 Hu, window level -650 - -500 Hu).

3.7　Diagnostic Guidelines of COVID-19

3.7.1　The Applicable Objects

Patients who have fever of unknown cause (body temperature $>$ 37.3℃) or acute respiratory infection of unknown cause, if they have contact history of traveling and living in Wuhan, or contact history of local confirmed or suspected patients, should be selected as the key screening groups.

3.7.2　Method of Examination

DR or CT examination. The first choice is CT.

3.7.3　Confirmation of Imaging Diagnosis

3.7.3.1　No abnormalities were Found in CT Examination (preferred) or DR Examination

Routine reports were performed, and relevant clinical examinations were recommended. No abnormalities were excluded and diagnosed after 14 days' review.

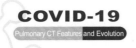
3.7.3.2 CT Examination (Preferred) or DR Examination Revealed Abnormalities

Lung CT or DR showed single or multiple small patch-shaped shadows, ground glass shadows with or without interstitial changes. The middle and lower lung fields and peripheral areas of both lungs were observed. In the progressive stage, multiple ground glass shadows and infiltration shadows were observed in both lungs

1. For the patients with the above typical imaging manifestations, the physician should review and report the critical value. If the imaging diagnosis is confirmed, it is recommended to do relevant laboratory tests in clinical practice to finally confirm the diagnosis.

2. For patients with atypical imaging performance, if the doctor on duty still considers suspected COVID-19 as the first choice, they will give a suspected diagnosis, review and report the critical value, and suggest improving the relevant clinical examination.

3. For patients with atypical imaging performance, if the doctor on duty isn't sure, please consult the leader or deputy leader of the chest group for consultation. If the diagnosis is still not possible, please consult the director of the department. If the diagnosis is suspected, follow option 2 above; if the diagnosis is considered to be excluded, follow option 1 (Fig. 3-7-1).

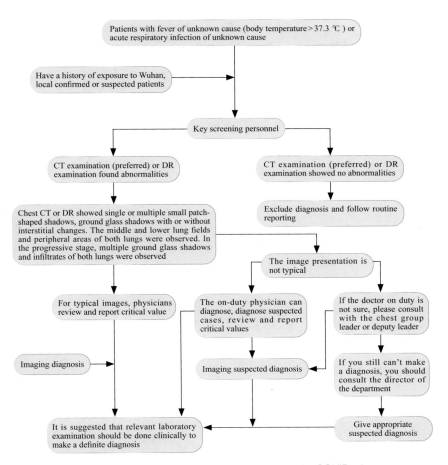

Fig. 3-7-1　Radiology diagnostic procedures for COVID-19

4

Image Stage and Pathological Basis of COVID-19

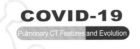

4.1 Imaging Staging of COVID-19

There is a lack of systematic radiological findings and case-control data. Based on the current clinical practice, CT manifestations of COVID-19 are recommended to be divided into four stages: early stage, progressive stage, severe stage and dissipation stage according to the extent and presentation of lesion involvement.

4.1.1 Early Stage

1. Distribution of lesions: mostly distributed in the middle and lower lobes, mostly under the pleura or interlobar fissure, or along the bronchovascular bundle distribution.

2. Number of lesions: often in both lungs.

3. Density of lesions: ①Ground-glass opacity (GGO) is more common in the lungs, thickening of the bronchial wall, thickening of the vascular shadow, lacked smooth in lung edge, slight thickening of the adjacent interlobar pleura; ②The range of lung consolidation is small, the air bronchogram sign of the bronchioles can be seen; ③The density of lesions is not uniform; ④GGO can exist alone or simultaneously with the consolidation.

4.Shape of lesions: irregular or fan-shaped is more common, can also be patchy or round, generally does not involve the lung segment.

5.Extrapulmonary manifestations: no underlying disease, no mediastinal lymph node enlargement, no pleural effusion.

4.1.2 Progressive Stage

1. Distribution of lesions: the distribution area is increased and enlarged, mainly under the pleura, and can involve multiple pulmonary lobes.

2. Shape of lesions: irregular, fan-shaped, or wedge-shaped.

3. Number of lesions: multiple lesions in both lungs.

4. Range of lesions: the lesion scope is enlarged, and multiple new lesions are common, which are scattered in multiple foci, patchy and even diffuse, and can be fused into large areas, with bilateral asymmetry. The density shadow or consolidation shadow of the original GGO can also be fused or partially absorbed. After fusion, the lesion scope and shape often change and are not completely distributed along the bronchovascular bundle.

5. Extrapulmonary manifestations: Pleural effusion or mediastinal lymph node enlargement is present in a few cases.

4.1.3 Severe Stage

1. The disease progressed further, with diffuse consolidation and uneven density in both lungs, with air bronchogram sign and tracheobronchial dilatation. The non-consolidation area may show patchy GGO, and most of the lungs show "white lung" appearance when affected. At 48 hours, the lesion area increased by 50%, mainly consolidation, combined with GGO, air bronchogram sign, multiple strip shadow.

2. Extrapulmonary presentation: interlobar pleura and bilateral pleura are often thickened, with a small amount of pleural effusion, showing free dissipation or local wrapping.

4.1.4 Absorption Stage

1. The absorption phase usually occurs about 1 week after the onset of the disease, in which the lesion scope is reduced, the density is reduced, the lung consolidation gradually disappears, the exudate is absorbed or organized, the lesions can be completely absorbed, part of

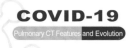
the residual strip shadow.

2. The improvement of the disease on imaging is usually later than the clinical symptoms, some lesions increase in scope, or new lesions appear.

4.2   Pathological Basis of COVID-19

4.2.1   Etiological Characteristics

COVID-19 belongs to the genus β, with an envelope, and the virus particles are round or oval, often polymorphic, with a diameter of 60-140 nm, and their genetic characteristics are related to acute respiratory distress syndrome coronavirus (SARS-CoV) There is a clear difference between the coronavirus (MERS-CoV) associated with the Middle East Respiratory Syndrome (MERS). Current research shows that the homology with bat SARS-like coronavirus (bat-SL-CoVZC45) is over 85%. When isolated and cultured in vitro, 2019-nCoV can be found in human respiratory tract epithelial cells in about 96 hours, while isolation and culture in Vero E6 and Huh-7 cell lines takes about 6 days (Fig. 4-2-1).

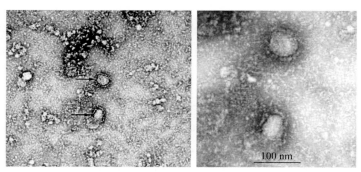

Fig. 4-2-1   Image by a novel coronavirus(↑) electron microscope
(Form: https://new.qq.com/omn/20200124/20200124A0AXVQ00.html)

4.2.2 Anatomical Histopathology

Studies have shown that: histological examination showed bilateral diffuse alveolar injury with mucous exudation of cell fibers (Fig. 4-2-2); obvious alveolar epithelial detachment and pulmonary hyaline membrane formation in the right lung tissue, suggesting ARDS (Fig. 4-2-2A), the left lung tissue showed pulmonary edema and pulmonary hyaline membrane formation, suggesting early ARDS (Fig. 4-2-2B), and both lymphocytes in the interstitial mononuclear cells can be seen in both lungs Sexual infiltration; multinucleated giant cells and atypically enlarged alveolar cells appear in the alveolar cavity. Among them, atypically enlarged alveolar cells have large nuclei, amphiphilic cytoplasmic granules and obvious nucleoli, showing viruses viral cytopathic-like changes; no obvious intranuclear or intracytoplasmic viral inclusions were found; the pathological features of COVID-19 are very similar to those of SARS and MERS coronavirus infections.

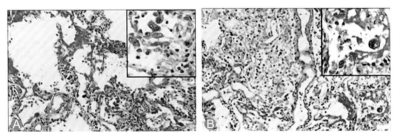

Fig. 4-2-2   Pathological features of the right(A) and left(B) lungs of a patient with COVID-19(HE staining, ×10)

4.2.3 Features of Imaging Pathology

The secondary lobule is the basic structural unit of the lung. It is polygonal, surrounded by connective tissue, and contains alveoli. It mainly includes the lobular core, lobular periphery, lobular interval, and lobular parenchyma(Fig. 4-2-3).

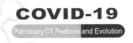
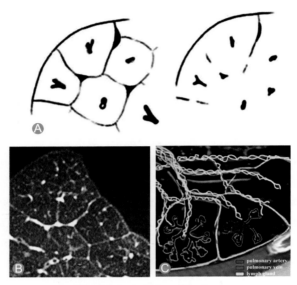

Fig. 4-2-3　Lobules of the lung

A. Schematic diagram of normal pulmonary lobules; B. HRCT of pulmonary lobules; C. Schematic diagram of interlobular septum

The core of the lobule mainly includes the bronchiole and the accompanying pulmonary artery, followed by the lymphatic vessel, and is surrounded by interstitial (the connective tissue sheath). The periphery of the leaflet travels at the junction of the leaflet (located around the leaflet). The content is the same as the core of the leaflet. It is the core of the other leaflets. It mainly includes the bronchioles and accompanying arterioles, followed by the lymphatic vessels, which are surrounded by the interstitial (the connective tissue sheath).

The leaflet is connected to the connective tissue plate, which surrounds the segmented lung lobule, mainly including veins and lymphatic vessels.

The lobular parenchyma is dominated by alveoli (Fig. 4-2-3).

Air bronchogram sign: the pathogen invades the epithelial cells, causing inflammatory thickening and swelling of the bronchial wall, but does not block the bronchiole (Fig. 4-2-4A).

Ground-glass opacity: the pathogen invaded the bronchial and alveolar epithelium and reproduced in the epithelial cells, causing non-bloody exudation. The exudation contains inflammatory cells such as affected epithelial cells and lymphocytes, and forms a membrane with protein and cellulose. The membrane is half thin and half thick, thicker than the initial bacterial phase and thinner than alveolar hemorrhage. Pathology: partial air cavity filling, alveolar interstitial thickening or slightly thickened interlobular septa, partial alveolar collapse and increased capillary blood volume(Fig. 4-2-4B and Fig. 4-2-4C).

Consolidation: the air chamber is fully filled (Fig. 4-2-4D and Fig. 4-2-4E).

"Honeycomb sign": balloon polymerization, representing fibrosis. Pathology: the transverse cut of tracheal bronchiectasis, and the surrounding fibrosis leads to the dilatation of the air cavity (Fig. 4-2-4F and Fig. 4-2-4G).

"Crazy paving pattern": GGO is accompanied by interlobular septa and lobular thickening, indicating that both the interstitium and the lumen are involved (Fig. 4-2-4H and Fig. 4-2-4I).

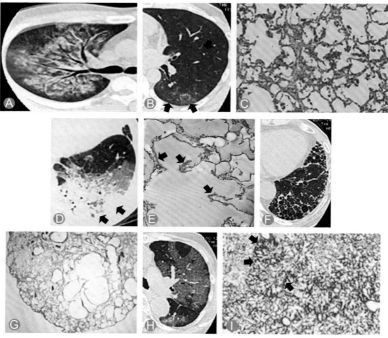

Fig. 4-2-4   A. Manifestation of air bronchogram sign; B. Subpleural GGO of the left lung(↑); C. Subpleural GGO of the left lung (HE staining, ×10); D. Consolidation shadows of the left lower lung(↑) E.Pathogenic manifestations of the left lower lung consolidation shadows (HE staining, ×100); F. "Honeycomb sign" of the left lung; G. Pathological findings of left lung "honeycomb sign" (HE staining, ×10); H. "Crazy paving pattern" of the left lung(↑); I. Pathological manifestations of "Crazy paving pattern" of left lung (HE staining,× 10)

4.3   Clinical and Pathological Changes of COVID-19

Studies have shown that: after the virus invaded the human body, on the one hand, due to the invasion of cells, leading to tissue and organ damage in the human body, resulting in the corresponding functional damage; On the other hand, human immune cells will release various cytokines, free radicals and other substances to attack the invading virus, thus causing organ damage. Especially, excessive immune response will lead to serious organ damage. Although viral pneumonia caused by various viruses may have various manifestations, it generally presents as several possible changes in lung injury, including diffuse alveolar injury, acute bronchitis, organized pneumonia and diffuse interstitial pneumonia.

Early-stage: the virus enters the airway to stimulate the respiratory tract and causes reflex cough, but has not yet caused alveolar effusion verification, only presenting acute interstitial inflammation, with alveolar septitis cell infiltration mainly consisting of small and medium lymphocytes. The patient presents with fever, dry cough and other symptoms clinically.

Acute effusion stage: histologically, diffuse alveolar epithelial injury, regional pulmonary edema, and the formation of part of the transparent membrane in the alveolar cavity. Virus inclusion bodies may be found in the infected alveolar epithelium. Clinically, patients may have symptoms such as breath suffocation and sputum cough, and multiple small patchy shadows can be seen on imaging examination (Fig. 4-3-1A and Fig. 4-3-1B).

Desquamation stage: the alveolar epithelium, the terminal bronchiole epithelium, and the basement membrane, which are inherent or proliferative, disintegrate and fall off into the alveolar cavity. Some of the epithelial cells are necrotic or apoptotic and are mixed with inflammatory exudate, resulting in the alveolar cavity being completely filled with inflammatory exudate and necrotic matter (Fig. 4-3-1C and Fig. 4-3-1D). At this time, patients will have obvious dyspnea and even ARDS, causing a series of acid-base imbalance and electrolyte imbalance in vivo. Especially for middle-aged and elderly

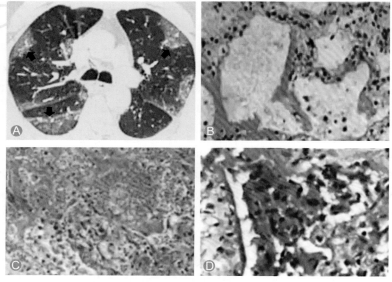

Fig. 4-3-1   Lung CT image and pathological changes of COVID-19

A. Double lung multiple grinding shadows(↑); B. Formation of clear membrane in alveolar cavity(HE staining, ×100); C. Alveolar hemorrhage and exudation(HE staining, ×10); D. Epithelial cells proliferating and exfoliating in alveolar space(HE staining, ×20)

patients with basic diseases, they often die due to respiratory and circulatory failure. The imaging findings were "white lung".

Repair stage: after active treatment or improvement of the patient's own resistance, the lesions will change into the proliferative and repair stage, manifested as hyperplasia of alveolar epithelial and terminal bronchiolar epithelial, early fibrosis and alveolar glomerulonephritis prototype, etc.

5

CT Features of the Early Stage of COVID-19

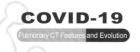
The early lesions of COVID-19 are mostly located in the periphery of the lung or under the pleura, mainly in the lower lobe of the lungs; often the lungs are multiple lesions, and the single lesion is rare; the lesions are irregular, fan-shaped, and flaky or round The lesion generally does not affect the entire lung segment; the density of the lesion is uneven, and it is more common with GGO, in which thickened blood vessels and bronchial passages can be seen, with or without grid-like thickening of the leaflet interval. In mild cases, the lesions mostly exist as ground glass density shadows. In severe cases, the consolidation can be combined, or the main changes can be seen, in which air bronchogram sign can be seen; the long axis of the lesion is parallel to the pleura. Those without other lung diseases generally did not have mediastinal and hilar lymphadenopathy, and no pleural thickening or pleural effusion were seen.

5.1 Typical CT Manifestations of Mild Cases of COVID-19 in an Early Stage

5.1.1 Distribution, Shape, and Number of Lesions

It is often a multifocal lesion of the lungs, which is located in the peripheral zone of the lungs or under the pleura, and is more common in the lower lobe of both lungs; the lesions are more irregular and fan-shaped (Fig. 5-1-1).

5.1.2 Ground-glass Opacity

A hazy image of increased lung density with high density pulmonary vascular shadows, suggesting alveolar exudate, alveolar wall swelling, or septal inflammation. The GGO lesions in the lung may be combined with thickening of blood vessels, interlobular thickening or air bronchogram (Fig. 5-1-2).

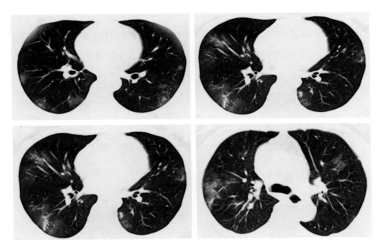

Fig.5-1-1　Multiple patchy, fan-shaped ground glass high density shadows were seen below the pleura in bilateral lobes with unclear boundaries

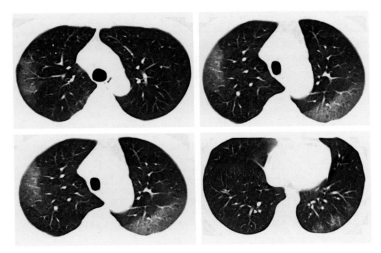

Fig.5-1-2　The patchy ground glass shadow is distributed in the subpleural area of bilateral pulmonary lobes

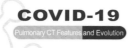
5.1.3 "Crazy Paving Pattern"

High-resolution CT shows that the thickening of interlobular septal and interlobular septal lineaments are superimposed on an opaque ground glass background, similar in shape to an irregular paving stone (Fig. 5-1-3).

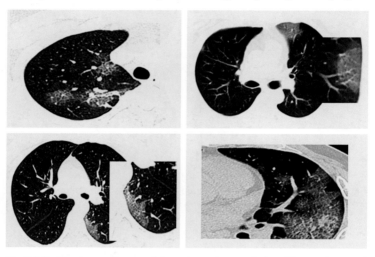

Fig.5-1-3   The two pulmonary lobes showed ground glass-like patches, and the interlobular septa thickened, showing a "crazy paving pattern", and the thickened vascular shadow could be seen

5.1.4   Air Bronchogram Sign

Air bronchogram sign refers to the phenomenon that when the lung is consolidated, the air bronchi contained in the consolidated lung tissue shows a shadow of dendritic low density(Fig. 5-1-4).

5.1.5   Vascular Thickening Sign

Vessel thickening sign refers to the thickened vessel shadow in or around the GGO(Fig. 5-1-5).

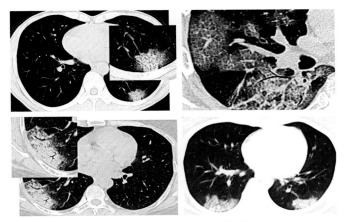

Fig.5-1-4　Patchy ground glass or high density shadow can be seen in the bilateral pulmonary lobes, the air bronchogram sign can be seen in the lung lobe, and some of the pavement stone sign and thickening blood vessel shadow can be seen

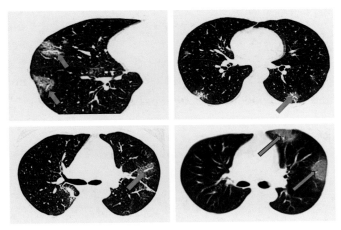

Fig.5-1-5　The two pulmonary lobes showed frosted vitreous plaques(⬆), and the thickened blood vessels in or around them were frosted vitreous plaques

5.1.6　Subpleural Line

The long axis of the lesion is parallel to the pleura, suggesting that the

lesion first involves the cortical lung tissue(Fig. 5-1-6).

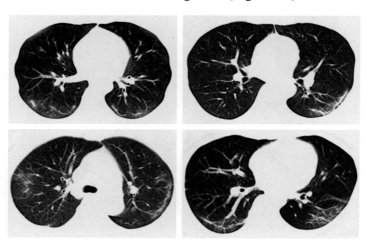

Fig.5-1-6   Below the pleura of the lower lobes of both lungs is an arcuate density parallel to the pleura

5.1.7   Negative Sign

Patients without other lung diseases generally have no hilum, mediastinal lymph node enlargement or pleural effusion.

5.2   CT Manifestations of Severe Cases of COVID-19 in an Early Stage

In the early stage, severe lesions of COVID-19 are more extensive than mild ones, mainly with GGO and consolidation shadows, which are still common under the pleura. Thickened blood vessels and "crazy paving pattern" are often seen in GGO lesions, as well as air bronchogram sign(Fig. 5-2-1).

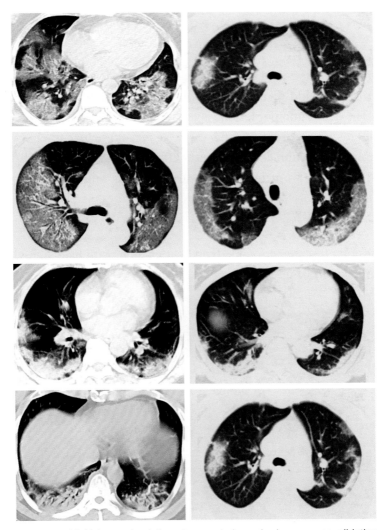

Fig.5-2-1   Multiple patchy, falloped ground glass shadows or consolidation shadows were seen in the bilateral pulmonary lobes. The lesions were mainly distributed under the pleura. Thickening of interlobular septa was seen in the ground glass like lesions, presenting a "crazy paving pattern", and thickening of blood vessels and air bronchogram sign were also seen

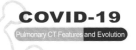

5.3 CT Manifestations of Atypical Cases of COVID-19 in an Early Stage

In both mild cases and severe cases, the single lesion is rare, with a few similar round or nodular lesions, and halo sign or reverse halo sign. The distribution of lesions is not mainly subpleural, but randomly distributes or according to the vascular and bronchial tracts. A few cases may be combined with pleural effusion. Therefore, it is difficult to differentiate from lung adenocarcinoma or other types of viral pneumonia.

5.3.1 Shape of Lesions

The lesion presented a rounded, nodular change, with halo sign visible in some nodules(Fig. 5-3-1).

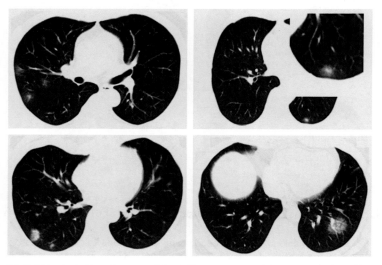

Fig.5-3-1 In both pulmonary lobes, there were nodular ground glass like high-density shadows of different sizes, halo sign was seen around some lesions, and the boundary of some lesions was clear

5.3.2 Nature of the Lesions

The lesions were mainly consolidation and a few of them had small voids(Fig. 5-3-2).

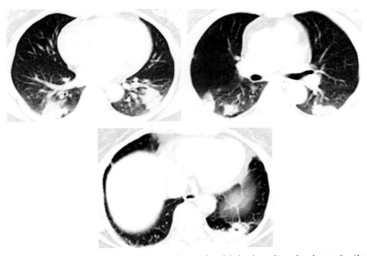

Fig.5-3-2　There are patchy and patchy high-density shadows in the subpleural lobes of the double pulmonary lobes, with unclear boundaries, small cavitation shadows can be seen in some lesions

5.3.3 Distribution of Lesions

The single lesion is rare and distributes randomly or according to the vascular bronchus(Fig. 5-3-3).

5.3.4 Complications

Only a few lesions may be associated with pleural effusion(Fig. 5-3-4).

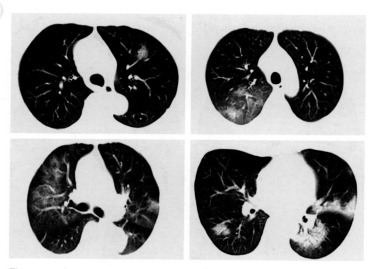

Fig.5-3-3　Single or multiple patchy ground glass or high density shadows were seen in the double pulmonary lobes. Some lesions were distributed along the vascular and bronchial tracts, while others were fan-shaped, with blurred boundaries

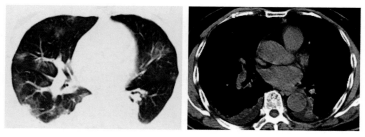

Fig.5-3-4　Multiple patchy ground glass shadows were seen in bilateral pulmonary lobes with blurred boundaries. A small amount of effusion was seen in the thorax on both sides, accompanied by a slight underexpansion of the lower lobe of both lungs

6

CT Manifestations of COVID-19 in an Advanced Stage

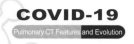

The progression period of COVID-19 is generally occurs 5-8 days after the onset of initial symptoms. At this stage, the infection quickly aggravates and spreads to the bilateral lung lobes, showing a diffuse GGO, and some lesions are consolidated. GGO coexist with real shadows or stripe shadows, and may be accompanied by thickening of the leaflet interval.

6.1 Typical CT Manifestations of Mild Cases of COVID-19 in an Advanced Stage

Bilateral lobes are often involved and subpleural distribution is asymmetric. Consolidation coexisted with GGO, and the consolidation lesions increased in the early stage, air bronchogram sign, halo sign, and reverse halo sign can be seen in the consolidation(Fig. 6-1-1-Fig. 6-1-4).

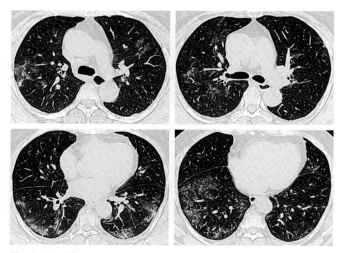

Fig. 6-1-1　The patient was a 61-year-old woman with fever, cough and chest tightness for 5 days, the picture was of progressive mild pulmonary CT, showing multiple ground-glass density shadows (partial subsolid) in both lungs

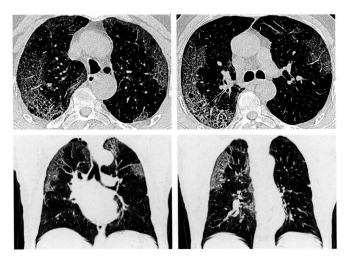

Fig. 6-1-2　A 70-year-old male was admitted to the hospital with cough and fever for 1 day. CT scan demonstrated that there were subpleural GGO and local stromal lesions in both lungs

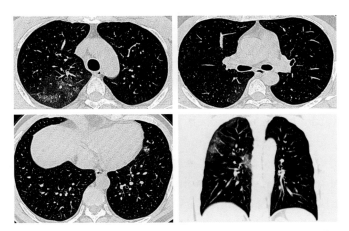

Fig. 6-1-3　The patient, a 43-year-old male, was feverish for half a day. The pulmonary CT of progressive mild disease is shown in the upper lobe of the right lung, the lower lobe and the tongue segment of the upper lobe of the left lung(multi-lobe involved)

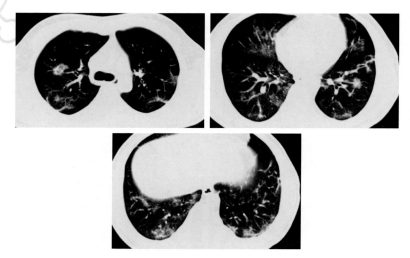

Fig. 6-1-4　The patient, a 39-year-old man, is shown with advanced mild disease CT, presenting multiple ground-glass plaques in both lungs, with reverse halo sign in the lesion in the right lung

6.2　Typical CT Manifestations of Severe Cases of COVID-19 in an Advanced Stage

The distribution area of the lesions is increased, mainly distributed under the pleura, which can involve multiple pulmonary lobes, can progress from the outer periphery of the lung to the center. The fusion of some lesions is enlarged and the density is increased, which is irregular, wedge-shaped, or fan-shaped; some lesions can be multifocal and fused in large areas, showing bilateral asymmetry. Broncho-vascular bundle thickening or multifocal consolidation of soft tissue density shadow under pleura, the lesion progresses and changes rapidly, showing subsegmental atelectasis, combined with pulmonary fibrosis, A few cases present pleural effusion(Fig. 6-2-1-Fig. 6-2-12).

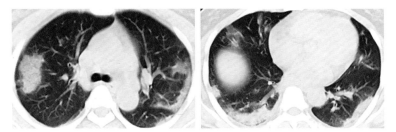

Fig. 6-2-1　The patient is a 52-year-old woman with cough and fever for 10 days. The picture was of advanced severe lung CT, showing multiple ground glass and consolidation shadows in both lungs, with air bronchiologram sign

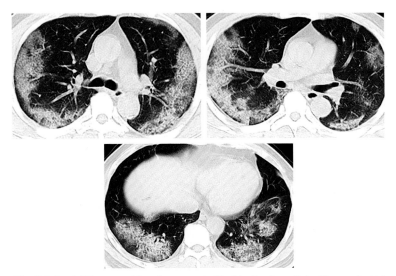

Fig. 6-2-2　A 55-years-old male was admitted to the hospital with cough and fever for 8 days, the picture is of advanced severe lung CT, showing GGO or consolidation shadows in both lungs, air bronchogram sign, and lesions involving multiple lobes

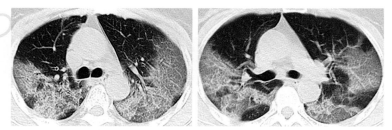

Fig. 6-2-3　A 65-year-old woman was admitted to the hospital due to fever and cough for 11 days. CT scan showed a large area of GGO on both sides of the pleura and thickened vascular shadow in some lesions

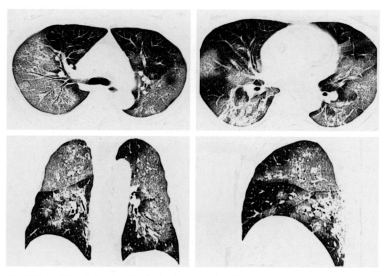

Fig. 6-2-4　The patient, a 56-year-old male, had fever and cough for half a day. CT scan of advanced severe lung showed GGO, consolidation shadow or cable shadow in both lungs, multiple pulmonary lobes involved, air bronchogram sign was visible, blood vessels in the lesions thickened, pulmonary fibrosis could be seen in the lesions located in the lower lobe of both lungs

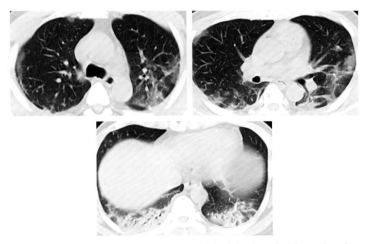

Fig. 6-2-5 A 37-year-old male patient visited the hospital for 1 day due to fever. CT scan showed multiple plaques and patchy shadows in both lungs, and subpleural multifocal lung consolidation

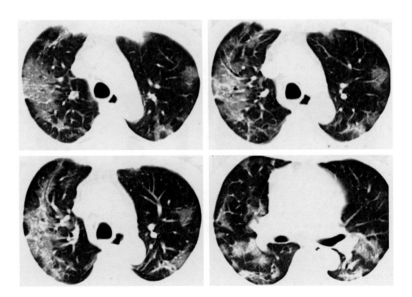

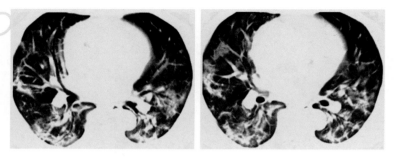

Fig. 6-2-6　This is a 54 year old male patient, whose CT scan showed advanced severe lung, presenting multiple ground glass plaques (partial subsolid) in both lungs, with air bronchogram sign, and nodules and striations in the lesions of the lower lobe of both lungs

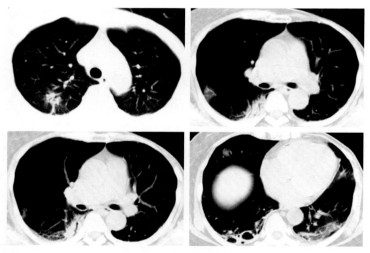

Fig. 6-2-7　Female patient, 62 years old, whose CT scan showed advanced severe lung, presenting multifocal subpleural lung consolidation, local lesions with fibrosis

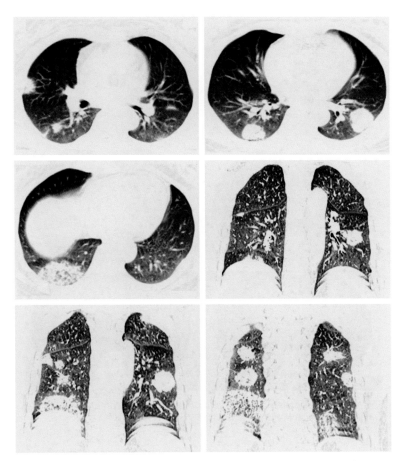

Fig. 6-2-8 This is a 45-year-old female patient with advanced severe pulmonary CT scan, showing increased lesions distribution, expanded fusion of some lesions, increased density, and "mass-like" changes

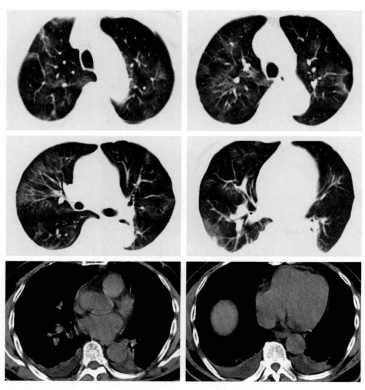

Fig. 6-2-9　The patient was 75 years old male. CT scan showed a wide range of lesions and a small amount of pleural effusion

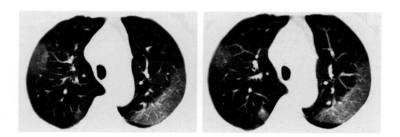

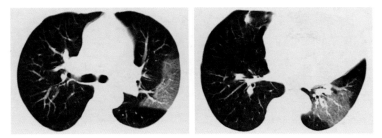

Fig. 6-2-10　The patient, a 74-year-old male, is shown with advanced severe pulmonary CT scan, showing increased lesion distribution areas, predominant subpleural distribution, and thickened vascular and bronchial bundles

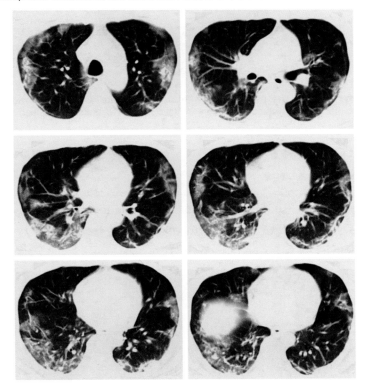

Fig. 6-2-11　The patient is a 47-year-old female with advanced severe pulmonary CT, presenting with subpleural focal plaques and nodules with fibrosis. The vascular and bronchial bundles were thickened with local interstitial changes

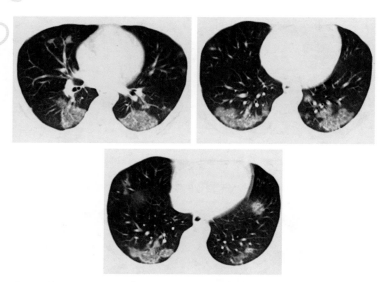

Fig. 6-2-12   The patient was a 34-year-old male. CT scan showed multifocal GGO with consolidation and thickening of vessels in the lesion

6.3   Atypical CT manifestations of COVID-19 in an Advanced Stage

The lesions are scattered patches, cord shadows, or patchy solid shadows, which are difficult to distinguish from other types of pneumonia(Fig. 6-3-1 and Fig. 6-3-2).

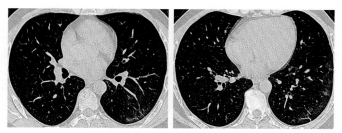

Fig. 6-3-1   A 41-year-old man was treated for fever and cough for 3 days. CT examination revealed plaques and streaks in the lower lobe of the left lung

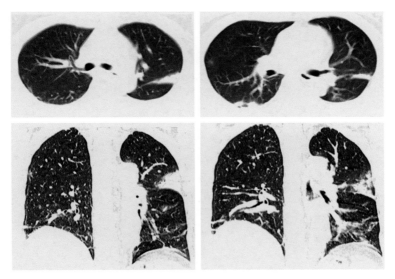

Fig. 6-3-2　A 35-year-old female patient, presented with a CT scan of the left lower lobe of the lung with pulmonary consolidation

7

CT Features of COVID-19 in Peak Period

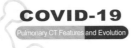
In peak period of COVID-19 (occurs 9-13 days after the initial symptoms), the CT manifestations of the lung are more stable than that of the progressive stage. The size, number, density and distribution range of the lesions in the lung reach the peak value. The original ground-glass density increases and generally progresses to mixed density or consolidation foci. CT scanning during this period may show mixed GGO, "crazy paving pattern", consolidation, etc., consolidation and air bronchogram sign are common, with or without fibrosis changes, etc. The pathology suggested diffuse alveolar injury with mucinous exudation of fine cells.

The CT findings of mild and severe patients at their peak vary in degree.

7.1 Typical CT Manifestations of Mild Cases of COVID-19 in Peak Period

The lesions of mild patients are limited, which can involve two lungs or one lung, usually occurring under the pleura. The lesions are mostly GGO or mixed density shadow with different sizes, which can be accompanied by a small range of consolidation and fibrosis trend, and the long axis is mostly parallel to the pleura(Fig. 7-1-1-Fig. 7-1-7).

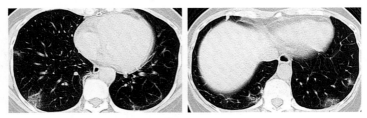

Fig. 7-1-1　The patient was a 45-year-old female with fever and cough for 2 days and a history of contact with the confirmed patient, the pulmonary CT scan on the 6th day after the onset of the disease showed multiple GGO in the subpleural lungs of both lungs, more visible in the following lobes, accompanied by thickened blood vessels and thickened interlobular septa

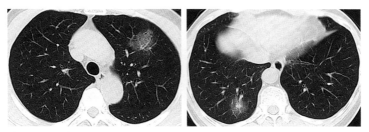

Fig. 7-1-2 The patient, a 69-year-old male, had fever and cough for 1 day and had contact history with the confirmed patient, the pulmonary CT scan on the 7th day after the onset of the disease showed GGO in the lower lobe of the right lung and the upper lobe of the left lung, accompanied by thickened blood vessels and thickened interlobular septa

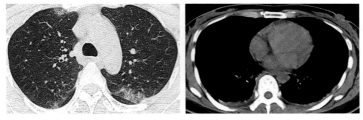

Fig. 7-1-3 The patient was a 45-year-old female with fever and cough for 4 days and a history of contact with the confirmed patient, the pulmonary CT scan on the 8th day showed multiple ground-glass density shadows near the oblique fissure of both lungs and a small amount of fluid on both sides of the chest

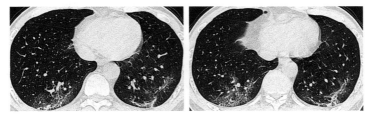

Fig. 7-1-4 Male, 43 years old, visited the hospital one day after the fever and had a history of contact with the confirmed patient, the pulmonary CT scan on the 7th day after onset showed multiple patchy, GGO with fibrosis trend in the lower lobe of both lungs, partial bronchiectasis and thickening of interlobular septa

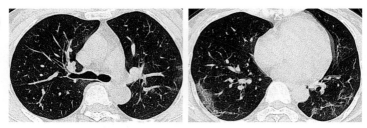

Fig. 7-1-5　A 48-year-old female, who went to the hospital for 1 day due to fever, had a confirmed patient's contact history. The pulmonary CT scan on the 12th day showed multiple ground-glass density shadows with fibrosis trend in both lungs, partial bronchiectasis and thickening of interlobular septa

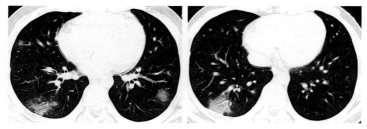

Fig. 7-1-6　The patient was a 12-year-old male with no symptoms and had a history of contact with the confirmed patient. The pulmonary CT scan on the 2nd day after the onset showed multiple GGO in both lungs distributed along the bronchovascular bundles with the presence of empty bronchus

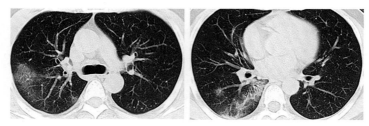

Fig. 7-1-7　The patient was a 43-year-old male with fever and cough for 1 day and had a history of contact with the confirmed patient. The pulmonary CT scan on the 8th day after the onset, which showed that there were multiple GGO in the right lung accompanied by partial consolidation

7.2 Typical CT Manifestations of Severe Cases of COVID-19 in Peak Period

Diffuse lesions in both lungs are more common, the disease progressed rapidly, and the range of lesions can increased by 50% within 48 hours. If more than 1/2 of the lung field is occupied by lesions, "white lung" appears. The main feature of the lesion is consolidation, which is associated with GGO and can be accompanied by multiple lobar shadows. Usually combined with other diseases, and the condition is critical(Fig. 7-2-1-Fig. 7-2-10).

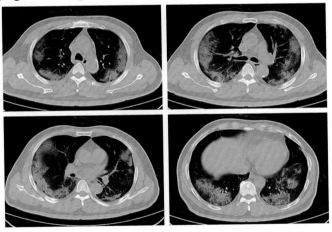

Fig. 7-2-1　The 56-year-old male patient had a history of contact with the confirmed patient, and the main symptoms are fever and dry cough. The CT scan of the lungs on the 10th day showed ground-glass density shadows and "crazy paving pattern", which are widely distributed in various lobes, especially subpleural

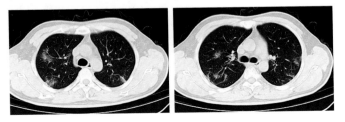

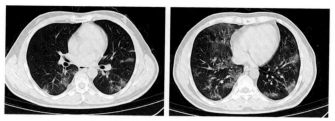

Fig. 7-2-2　The patient was a 39-year-old male who lived in Wuhan for a long time. The main symptoms were fever (38.5 °C) and dry cough. The pulmonary CT on the 17th day showed GGO, flake shadow or strip shadow

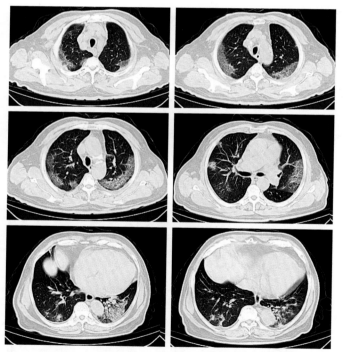

Fig. 7-2-3　The 54-year-old male patient had a history of contact with the diagnosed patient and had CT images on the 12th days after onset. The main signs were GGO, interlobular septal thickening, and stripy shadow. The lesion range was subpleural and intrapulmonary

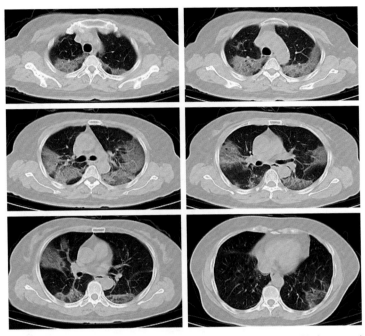

Fig. 7-2-4   The 45-year-old female patient lives in Wuhan with fever and dry cough as the main symptoms. The pulmonary CT image on the 15th days after onset showed GGO, "crazy paving pattern", strip shadow, and consolidation in the lower lobe of both lungs

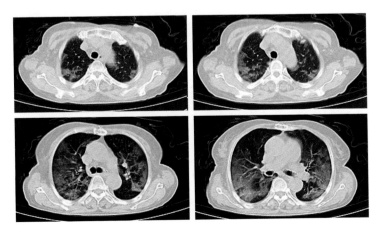

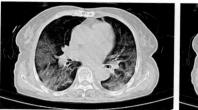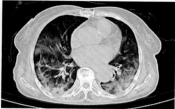

Fig. 7-2-5 The patient was a 70-year-old male with a history of exposure to the diagnosed patient, the main symptoms were fever, cough, and sputum, and combined with chronic bronchitis, emphysema. The pulmonary CT image on the 7th days after the onset of the disease showed "crazy paving pattern" and cable shadow, and the lesions were mainly subpleural

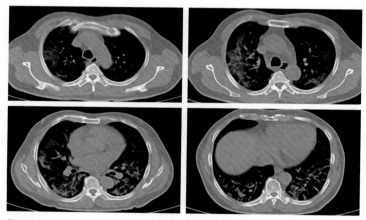

Fig. 7-2-6 The patient, a 30-year-old male who lived in Wuhan for a long time, presented with fever, chest tightness and diarrhea as the main symptoms. The CT appearance of the lung on the 4th day after the onset of the disease is shown here. The main signs are GGO, fiber cable shadow, and the lower lobe of the two lungs

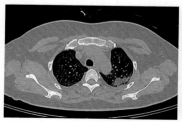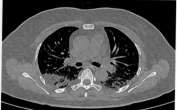

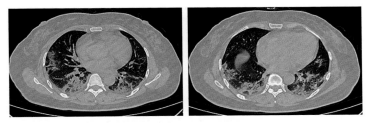

Fig. 7-2-7　The patient, male, 74 years old, lived in Wuhan, coughed, and coughed sputum without fever. The CT image of 18 days after onset, mainly presented with GGO, "crazy paving pattern" and left lower lobe with consolidation

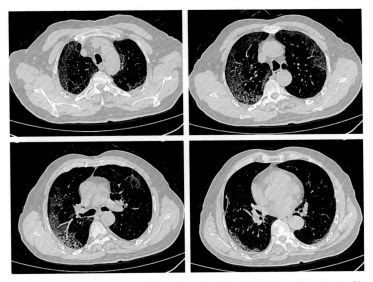

Fig. 7-2-8　The 65-year-old female patient had a history of contact with the confirmed patient and had CT images on the 10th days after onset presenting with GGO, "crazy paving pattern", and fiber cable shadow. The lesions involved subpleural and intrapulmonary, mainly in the upper lobe of both lungs

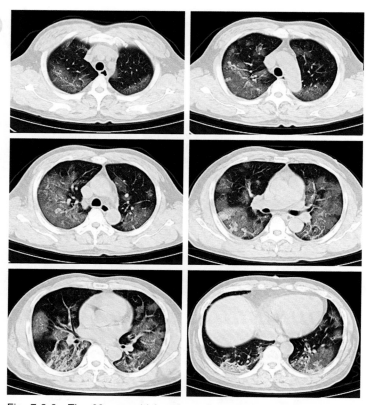

Fig. 7-2-9   The 68-year-old female patient came to the hospital with fever and diarrhea. CT images of the chest at 16 days after the onset were mainly shown as GGO, patch shadow, "crazy paving pattern", partial consolidation of the lower lobe of both lungs, and the lesion range was subpleural and intrapulmonary

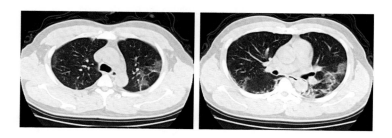

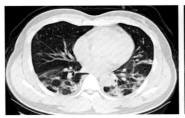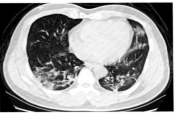

Fig. 7-2-10 The 56-year-old male patient had a history of contact with the confirmed patient and the main symptoms are fever and dry cough. This is the CT image of the lung at 7 days after onset of the disease. The main manifestations are ground glass density shadow, fiber cable shadow, and partial consolidation in the diffuse distribution of the two lungs

7.3 CT Features of Atypical COVID-19 in the Peak Period

Some patients with COVID-19 showed atypical chest CT manifestations in the peak period, mainly including the following conditions.

7.3.1 Distribution of Lesions

The lesions were only distributed in individual pulmonary lobes (segments), presenting single mixed density shadows or consolidation shadows, accompanied by air bronchogram sign, thickening of small vascular network and thickening of the interlobular septa (Fig. 7-3-1-Fig. 7-3-4).

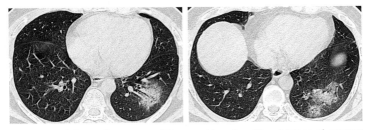

Fig. 7-3-1 The patient was a 38-year-old male with a history of contact with a confirmed patient. The main symptoms were fever and dry cough. The pulmonary CT on the 6th day after the onset presented with a single patch consolidation in the lower lobe of the left lung, accompanied by air bronchogram sign and thickening of the interlobular septum

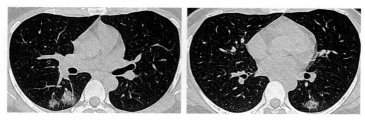

Fig. 7-3-2   A 33-year-old female patient with fever for 1 day had a history of contact with the confirmed patient. The pulmonary CT on the 11th day after onset, showed that multiple mixed GGO were seen in the subpleural area of the lower lobe of both lungs, and burring and lobules could be seen in some lesions

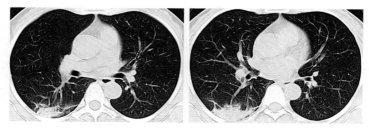

Fig. 7-3-3   The patient was a 55-year-old female with fever and cough for 1 day and a history of contact with the confirmed patient. The pulmonary CT on the 9th day showed a single subpleural mass consolidation shadow in the right lower lobe of the lung

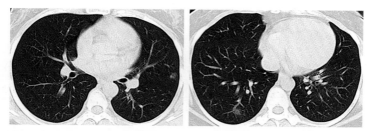

Fig. 7-3-4   Female, 34 years old, asymptomatic, with a confirmed patient history of exposure. The pulmonary CT on the 5th day after onset shows slight under the pleura of both lungs

7.3.2　Lesion Involvement

The lesions involve the internal and central areas of both lungs (Fig. 7-3-5 and Fig. 7-3-6).

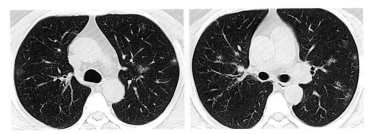

Fig. 7-3-5　The patient, a 48-year-old male, visited the doctor 3 days after fever and cough. The pulmonary CT on the 18th day showed multiple GGO in both lungs distributed along the bronchovascular bundles, mostly subpleural, with intrapulmonary involvement

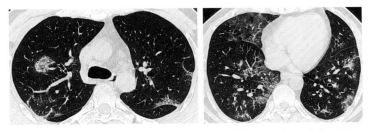

Fig. 7-3-6　The patient, a 39-year-old male, had fever and cough for 1 day. The CT scan of the lungs on the 14th day showed multiple GGO in both lungs with simultaneous involvement of the outer, middle and inner bands

8

CT Features of COVID-19 in Resolution Period

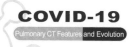
Resolution period is often occurs 10 days after the onset of pneumonia, some mild patients can be about 1 week in advance. Due to clinical infection control, lung lesions gradually absorbed, the scope of the lesions gradually reduced, lung consolidation gradually disappeared into GGO, and finally gradually disappeared or the remaining part of the cable shadow(Fig. 8-1-1-Fig. 8-1-4).

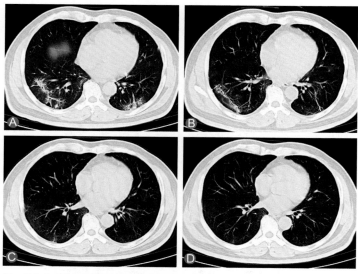

Fig. 8-1-1　The patient was a 56-year-old male with a history of exposure to COVID-19, had severe pneumonia. CT images on the 21st(A), 30th(B), 46th(C) and 65th(D) day after onset of the disease showed that the flaky shadow of the lower lobe of the two lungs was gradually absorbed, and the lesions in the left lower lobe of the lung disappeared on the 65th day of the disease, while the right lower lobe showed slight

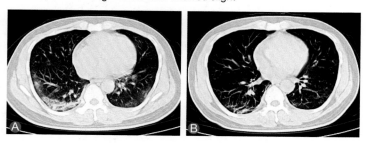

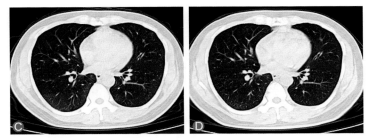

Fig. 8-1-2 A 41-years old male patient with heavy COVID-19, is living in Wuhan. The CT images on the 6[th](A), 9[th](B), 15[th](C), and 30[th](D) days after onset of COVID-19 showed that the consolidation shadow of the lower lobe of both lungs was gradually absorbed, evolved into strip shadow, and disappeared on the 30th day

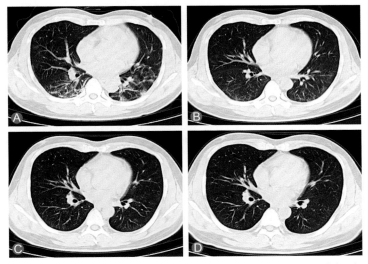

Fig. 8-1-3 A 37-years old male patient with heavy COVID-19, is living in Wuhan, The CT images on the 7[th](A), 16[th](B), 22[nd](C) and 36[th](D) day after onset of COVID-19 showed that multiple flaky shadows in both lungs were gradually absorbed and transformed into GGO. The changes in the two lung diseases disappeared on the 36th day

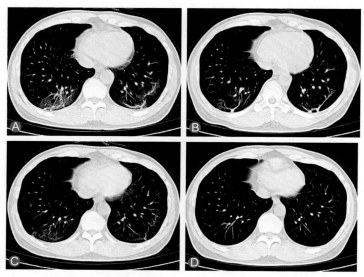

Fig. 8-1-4 A 43-years old male patient with mild COVID-19, is living in Wuhan, The CT images on the 7[th](A), 10[th](B), 17[th](C), and 46[th](D) days after onset of COVID-19 showed the flaky shadow, GGO, and "crazy paving pattern" of the lower lobe of the two lungs on the 7th day, "crazy paving pattern" basically disappeared on the 10th day, the flaky shadow evolved into GGO on the 17th day, and the lesions on both two lungs disappeared on the 46th day

参考文献

[1] CHAOLIN HUANG, YEMING WANG, XIN GWANG LI, et al. Clinical features of patients infected with 2019 novel coronavirus in Wuhan, China[J]. Lancet, 2020, 395（10223）: 497-506. DIO: 10.1016/S0140-6736（20）30183-5.

[2] QUN LI, XUHUA GUAN, PENG WU, et al. Early transmission dynamics in Wuhan, China, of novel coronavirus-infected pneumonia[J]. New England Journal of Medicine, 2020, 382（13）: 1199-1207. DIO: 10.1056/NEJMoa2001316.

[3] LAI C C, SHIH T P, KO W C, et al. Severe acute respiratory syndrome coronavirus 2（SARS-CoV-2）and corona virus disease-2019（COVID-19）: the epidemic and the challenges[J]. Int J Antimicrob Agents, 2020. DIO: 10.1016/jijantimicag. 2020.105924.

[4] XU X , CHEN P, WAN G J, et al. Evolution of the novel coronavirus from the on going Wuhan outbreak and modeling of its spike protein for risk of human transmission[J]. Science China Life Sciences, 2020, 63（3）: 457-460.

[5] HU BEN, ZENG LEI-PING, YANG XING-LOU, et al. Discovery of a rich gene pool of bat SARS-related coronaviruses provides new insights into the origin of SARS coronavirus[J]. PLoS pathogens, 2017, 13（11）: e100-166.

[6] ROUJIAN LU, XIANG ZHAO, JUAN LI, et al. Genomic characterization and epidemiology of 2019 novel coronavirus: implications for virus origins and receptor binding[J]. The Lancet, 2020（pre-publish）.

[7] ZHOU PENG, YANG XING-LOU, WANG XIAN-GUAN G, et al. A pneumonia outbreak associated with a new coronavirus of probable bat origin[J]. Nature, 2020, 5（7）: 270-273.

[8] ROUJIAN LU, XIANG ZHAO, JUAN LI, et al. Genomic characterisation and epidemiology of 2019 novel coronavirus: implications for virus origins and receptor binding[J]. Lancet, 2020, DIO: 10.1016/S0140-6736（20）30251-8.

[9] YANG YANG, QINGBIN LU, MINGJIN LIU, et al. Epidemiological and clinical features of the 2019 novel coronavirus outbreak in China[J]. Medrxiv Posted, 2020, 9（1）: 25-30.

[10] 国家中医药管理局办公室，国家卫生健康委办公厅. 关于印发新型冠状病毒肺炎诊疗方案（试行第七版）的通知 [EB/OL].（2020-03-03）[2020-04-09].

http://www.gov.cn/zhengce/zhengceku/2020-03/04/content_5486705.htm.

[11] ANNA-LUISE A，KATZENSTEIN M C. Diagnostic Atlas of Non-Neoplastic Lung Disease：A practical guide for surgical pathologists[J]. Demos Medical，2016.

[12] XU Z，SHIV L，WAN G Y J，et al. Pathological findings of COVID-19 associated with acute respiratory distress syndrome[J]. Lancet，2020.

[13] （美）葛内．赵绍宏，聂永康，主译．肺部高分辨率 CT[M]. 北京：人民卫生出版社，2010.

[14] 管汉雄，熊颖，申楠茜，等．武汉 2019 新型冠状病毒（2019-nCoV）肺炎的临床影像学特征初探 [J]. 放射学实践，2020，10（2）：1-6.

[15] 汪锴，康嗣如，田荣华，等．新型冠状病毒肺炎胸部 CT 影像学特征分析 [J]. 中国临床医学，2020，5（1）：27-31.

[16] 刘发明，丁惠玲，龚晓明，等．新型冠状病毒肺炎（COVID-19）的胸部 CT 表现与临床特点 [J]. 放射学实践，2020，3（1）：266-268.

[17] 龚晓明，李航，宋璐，等．新型冠状病毒肺炎（COVID-19）CT 表现初步探讨 [J]. 放射学实践，2020，3（6）：261-265.

[18] 史河水，韩小雨，樊艳青，等．新型冠状病毒（2019-nCoV）感染的肺炎临床特征及影像学表现 [J]. 临床放射学杂志，2020，7（6）：1-8.

[19] 陆雪芳，龚威，王莉，等．新型冠状病毒肺炎初诊临床特征及高分辨率 CT 影像表现 [J/OL]．中华放射学杂志，2020，54（2）：12-16. [2020-02-12]. http：// rs.yiigle.com/yufabiao/1180541.htm. DOI：10.3760/cma.j.issn.1005-1201.2020.0006.

[20] Suster S，Moran C A. Biopsy interpretation of the lung[J]. Lippincott Williams & Wilkins，a Wolters Kluwer，2013，10（3）：45-67.

[21] Anna-Luise A，Katzenstein M C. Diagnostic Atlas of Non-Neoplastic Lung Disease：A practical guide for surgical pathologists[J]. Demos Medical，2016，7（1）：10-28.

[22] 丁彦青．严重急性呼吸综合征的病理学及发病 机制 [J]. 解放军医学杂志，2003，28（6）：475-476.

[23] 申明识，尹彤，纪小龙．SARS 肺的病理鉴别诊断 [J]. 临床与实验病理学杂志，2003，19（4）：387-389.